ADVANCE PRAISE FOR *MOVEMENT MATTERS*

With *Movement Matters*, Katy Bowman has produced a thoughtful—and radical—treatise that is a must-read for those interested in their personal health…and the health of the body politic and planet. A stellar read.
—Rose Hayden-Smith, author of *Sowing the Seeds of Victory: American Gardening Programs of World War I*

I've spent almost twenty years talking to people about food and specifically why good food matters. I've made my case using biology and ecology, talking about our hunter-gatherer past. What I missed is all the movement that went into not just our food but also our lives. This is why movement matters—and fortunately for you, Katy Bowman has tackled this topic in a way that has never been done before.
—Robb Wolf, author of *The Paleo Solution*

In a civilization that strives to reduce movement to its barest minimum, and a culture that celebrates the leisure of the chair over the immersive experiences that truly nourish our bodies and souls, there is the voice of Katy Bowman. Her scientific approach, coupled with her deep understanding of the ancestral roots of our physiological needs, bridges the longstanding gap between the world of healthy movement and the advice of the medical and exercise science communities. Finally, we learn why movement matters, and that the answer lies not in the monotony of pointless exercise for its own sake, but rather in the exhilaration of move-ment as an expression of our very human
—Daniel Vitalis, host of the *ReWild Yours*

Understanding our role as human animals within the web of our ecosystem is critical in order to fully grasp what it means to exist. *Movement Matters* fully embraces all that I think we are failing to recognize—that our true selves are within the natural world, not above it.

—Diana Rodgers, RD, author of *The Homegrown Paleo Cookbook*

Katy Bowman is one of the world's leading experts on the ecology of human movement. She offers a timely and fascinating collection of essays that are designed to inspire a movement-based lifestyle— essential for our long-term survival as adaptive humans. A must-read for anyone who cares about their health.

—Angela Hanscom, author of *Balanced and Barefoot*

What a breath of fresh air! Katy Bowman, like her books, oozes originality and intelligence. In *Movement Matters*, she makes readers see how movement isn't something you do—it's something you are....The world, the fitness industry, and those of you at home aspiring for wellbeing will really benefit from Katy's life-enhancing information.

—Ellen Barrett, author of *The 28 Days Lighter Diet*

This is a compelling manifesto for an organic, natural movement lifestyle. Katy Bowman reminds us of essential principles about physiology, biology, life, movement, and even our connection to the world. Her insights are empowering and enlightening, and will help readers eliminate the unnecessary separation between their mindset and their physical behavior.

—Erwan Le Corre, founder of MovNat

This gorgeous book opens the door to a new way of thinking and being. Katy teaches us how each movement, no matter how small it may seem, matters. You can't help but want to become more active in every aspect of your life.
—Kristin Meekhof, author of *A Widow's Guide to Healing*

One of the unfortunate side effects of living in complex, modern societies is the distance we create from the natural world, leading us to forget how to live better with less and by keeping active. In her quest to resurrect this lost knowledge, Katy Bowman provides us with a survival roadmap to reclaim personal quality of life and a sustainable future for all. A must-read for anyone interested in living a happy, productive life on a habitable planet.
—Jason Lewis, author of *The Expedition*

Everyone should read this book.
—*Paleo Magazine*

In *Movement Matters*, Katy Bowman has taken a large and complex topic and made it more than just fathomable—the essays are an enjoyable exploration of movement and other features of human health viewed from a unique perspective. Rather than simply inspiring more exercise for personal health, she has formulated a beautiful argument that explains how recovering the large variety of movements Americans have outsourced to machines and workers in distant lands helps ecosystems (and the people who live within them)....*Movement Matters* is certainly worth the read.
—Arthur Haines, author of the *Ancestral Plants* volumes

ALSO BY KATY BOWMAN:

Simple Steps to Foot Pain Relief
Diastasis Recti
Whole Body Barefoot
Don't Just Sit There
Move Your DNA
Alignment Matters

MOVEMENT
matters

If the info in this book resonates with you and you would like to work with a Nutritious Movement-certified movement coach to help incorporate these ideas into your movement life,

email BRi at

shadowmovementcoaching@gmail.com

or visit

shadowmovementcoaching.com!

MOVEMENT
matters

Essays on:
MOVEMENT SCIENCE,
MOVEMENT ECOLOGY, AND
THE NATURE OF MOVEMENT

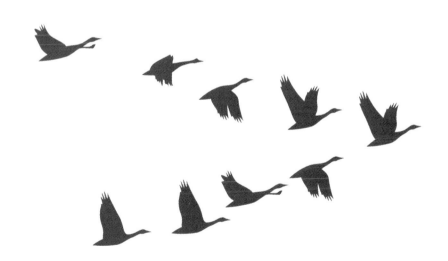

KATY BOWMAN

PROPRIOMETRICS
PRESS

Printed in the United States of America.
First Printing, 2016
ISBN-13: 978-1-943370-03-0
Library of Congress Control Number: 2016940676
Propriometrics Press: propriometricspress.com
Cover and Interior Design: Zsofi Koller, zsofikoller.com
Illustrations: Jillian Nicol
Author photos by J. Jurgensen Photography. All other photos by Michael Curran unless otherwise noted.

The information in this book should not be used for diagnosis or treat-ment, or as a substitute for professional medical care. Please consult with your healthcare provider prior to attempting any treatment on yourself or another individual.

Publisher's Cataloging-In-Publication Data
(Prepared by The Donohue Group, Inc.)
Names: Bowman, Katy. | Nicol, Jillian, illustrator.
Title: Movement matters : essays on: movement science, movement ecology and the nature of movement / Katy Bowman ; illustrations: Jillian Nicol.
Description: [Sequim, Washington] : Propriometrics Press, [2016] | Includes bibliographical references and index.
Identifiers: ISBN 978-1-943370-03-0 | ISBN 978-1-943370-04-7 (ebook)
Subjects: LCSH: Human locomotion. | Sedentary behavior. | Human ecology.
Classification: LCC RM725 .B693 2016 (print) | LCC RM725 (ebook) | DDC 615.82--dc23

For the man who, when I talk of muscles and sarcomeres, draws parallels to relationships among the universe, stars, planets, and people, and who, through example, taught me to take a walk every day. And for Roxana, who gets it.

CONTENTS

It's a pity we don't whistle at one another,
like birds. Words are misleading.

—HALLDOR LAXNESS

FOREWORD

The book you're holding is radical. Not because it contains powerful and almost peerless arguments for the personal adoption of physical movement, and not even because it illustrates how outsourcing your movement has far-reaching social, political, and ecological consequences. It is radical because when practiced, its movement-oriented messages enrich your life with an ineffable momentum that is as physical as it is existential. It will push you forward. I am testament to this. The messages here have completely changed my life for the better, and living them continues to change me—and my path—in ways I couldn't have imagined.

I was recently confronted with the fact that my greatest personal shortcoming is what I can only describe as a form of emotional paralysis. It is an immobility of sorts, an inability to foster deep connections with others, and ultimately myself, because I could never move to a place of vulnerability.

The revelation is still fresh, but I have a strong sense that this immobility is the symptom of a sedentary life—that the biomechanical, emotional, and psychical are much more interlinked than I can comprehend.

To date, I've lived a very fortunate life. I was raised by great parents, given a respectable education, and was systematically bestowed with opportunity after opportunity due to having won the existential lottery of being born a white, middle-class male.

This—along with hard work—enabled me to find relative success in early adulthood, and because of immaturity, misguidedness, and the influence of Western culture's obsession with materialism, I began to overindulge in creature comforts. And in this, I erred, gravely and almost to the grave. You see, by my early thirties I was achy, obese, and sick to the point of being hospitalized due to my chosen lifestyle.

But I didn't care at all; I actually scoffed at my worsening health. Why? Because I had transcended my social class and, in turn, felt like a joyous tourist to a previously unknown paradise. I couldn't get enough of enough—because in this mindset there would never be enough. I loved being shuttled around, I loved having takeout delivered to my desk, I loved outsourcing the laborious and the mundane.

And I was a complete and total idiot for it, for buying into this toxic lifestyle where capitalistic success is expressed as excess in everything but movement—earn more, move less. And while it's marketed to be desirable, it's very costly: Stasis and convenience are a prison cell where your body rots as your consciousness is captive for the length of your chosen sentence.

Oddly, I was beginning to sense this. But due to feelings of shame and embarrassment and the stinging memory of failed, half-assed attempts of trying to get fit in gyms, I couldn't muster up the courage to push open the cell's unlocked door. I just sat there apathetically.

But luckily, I was freed, randomly and unintentionally, by Katy

Bowman, a complete stranger I owe my life to.

In January 2015, at thirty-three years old, I was at my lowest point—ironically also my highest weight: pushing 260 pounds on a small 5′11″ frame. And I just happened to hear Katy talk about her field of study as a guest on a podcast. She has an impressive ability to distill complex biomechanics into layperson's terms, but beyond that, I was struck by how powerful and sensible her plea for varied movement was. It was so radical yet so logical, so modern yet so ancient. And above all else, it was fundamentally disruptive to countless norms and conventions that concern health, fitness, and lifestyle. It didn't just pique my interest—it pushed me to move. Specifically, to walk. I was inspired to take up a basic human function, as ridiculous as that sounds.

That winter, I began to walk, just a little bit each day, about an hour to and from work. At first it was purely functional, naturally fitting into my day while saving me the expense of public transit or taxi cabs. And because I did it in the dead of winter, I literally saved face "exercising" publicly, covering my face with a balaclava. I'd like to say it was enjoyable at first, but it really wasn't. It's embarrassing to admit, but movement was so foreign to my body that walking—as simple as it is—killed my feet, knees, and hips.

But my smartphone became an ally, enabling me to listen to my favorite music and podcasts, which made walking entertaining amidst the initial pain. And as my weight and pain decreased, my walking evolved from something functional to something also recreational, something I began to layer into my evenings and weekends. Furthermore, I found that I could stack my walks. I used walking to stitch together errands like shopping at different local grocers, which helped introduce dynamic loads into my walks. And I found I could use my smartphone to conduct calls and reply to emails using voice-to-text apps, all during my walks. Movement wasn't a detour from my work or career; it was a truly integrated part of it. All of this made the act of walking something I really enjoyed, and because of this, I challenged myself to walk 2,015 kilometers that year.

Luckily, I got hooked on walking before I grew tired of my music library and preferred podcasts. So the earbuds came out, and the city's sights and sounds came in. As the snow began to thaw that spring, so did I. And it was profound.

Walking is a slow thing—step by step, you just plod along. And because of its pace, you experience the world slowly, meditatively. You see and hear beautiful things: You hear marriage proposals, see acts of kindness, and get to interact with countless cute dogs. But you also experience terrible things, things you're literally forced to face daily, regularly, like staring into the faces of the dispossessed begging for money, or staring into the faces of young black men asking for your help as they're stopped and frisked by the police for no reason at all.

Witnessing these things made me think a lot, about my privilege and ultimately my purpose; in a way, walking streets, paths, and trails is akin to walking through the veins of a big global body that is more interconnected and interdependent than we generally realize. This made me reevaluate my relationship with movement—I realized I had been moving solely for my own self-improvement.

I had walked by so many problems. And it began to haunt me. I was walking in expensive sneakers past people with tattered shoes (or none altogether), walking in fancy wicking clothing to stay cool past people trying to stay warm, or going for a late-night walk to burn off an indulgent meal while walking past people who were starving. I wasn't naive enough to think I could dismantle systemic problems, but I couldn't in good conscience continue to walk by, either. So after walking a thousand kilometers, I began to distribute homemade (or hotel-room-made) sandwiches to hungry people on the streets, both in my community and in the many places and countries my job and personal travels took me to. In short, I reimagined my physical movement as social movement; I began to move beyond myself, to attempt to alleviate the suffering of others on my walks, albeit only temporarily.

By year's end, I had reached my goal of walking 2,015 kilometers. I lost a hundred pounds along the way, radically transforming and reclaiming my body. This brought me to a new baseline of health that let me vary my movement in new ways. I got into long-distance swimming, I free-lifted rocks of odd shapes and sizes on my family's farm, and I began to seriously practice boxing; the technique, foot-work, and shadowboxing of which have been physically liberating in indescribable ways. My physical changes are all cool, sure, but this was just a reset of sorts, and it pales in comparison to what walking and movement ultimately gave me.

In 2015 I actually walked more than my initial goal. I ended up walking over 5,800 kilometers and distributing a thousand sand-wiches along the way. I helped others, and did a tiny bit of good, but getting outside and moving outdoors did *me* a world of good: It helped me start the process of moving outside and beyond myself.

Katy writes in this book, "We are shaped by the forces we experi-ence." This is immensely true for me, first biomechanically but more importantly mentally and spiritually. Becoming a mover awakened my consciousness and inspired me to become an active participant in the world…rather than a secondhand observer of it through device screens, canned content, and the social media posts of others. Furthermore, it motivated me to start building the world I wanted to live in rather than accepting the world as it is.

As I approach my nine thousandth kilometer of walking, I often reflect on how far I've gone yet how little I've moved in other areas of my life and self. I don't question my initial reason for walking, but as Katy says, "There is always further to go." This is why I now try to stride towards the tribe—towards others—rather than to walk alone as I've done up until this point, solitarily, anonymously, and invisibly in crowds. Movement has connected me back to my physical self, and it's given me a greater momentum to connect with others. Today, that's why I move: because it brings me one step closer to new levels of love, vulnerability, and happiness. And to me, it's why this book matters. It's why movement matters.

BEN POBJOY

Toronto, ON
July 2016

INTRODUCTION

When we try to pick out anything by itself, we find it hitched to everything else in the Universe.

—JOHN MUIR

M ovement Matters. Not just movement—*your* movement. Not only to your physiology, but to those in your family and your community. Your movement matters, not only to those you see on a daily and yearly basis, but to humans elsewhere, that you've never met. Your movement matters to the forests and bees in your local area, and our culturally approved (and possibly demanded) sedentarism is responsible for much of the deforestation of the planet as well as slavery in other places.

You have a role in the ecosystem, and it's not a static position at the top of the food chain as you were taught. Your role is a dynamic one, critical to all the other living things on this planet.

I haven't always understood movement this way. This book is the result of me, a biomechanist—someone trained in the application

1

of mechanical laws to the movement and structure of living things—starting to think like an ecologist, and recognizing how movement is a part, a component, of our personal health, our communities, and our planet.

Ecology is a branch of biology that deals with the relationships of organisms to one another and to their physical surroundings. Movement ecology, then, is concerned with how an animal, in this case a human, moves, relative to other humans, relative to other species, and relative to their physical surroundings or environment or habitat.

Ten years ago you could have asked me, "What's the right way to walk?" and I could have given you the biomechanist's answer, including at what point heel strike and toe off should happen, which muscles should contract a lot and which should work in the background, and which shoes contain the features "best for the body." And that would have been my final answer, an answer stemming from my experience in the movement lab and exposure to thousands of research articles on data collected from people with various injuries and how they walked, and which corrective exercises improved their gait, and so on.

Today if you asked me, "What's the right way to walk?" I'd say that walking is a category of movements, not a single pattern—which means there is no single right way, only different ways that result in different outcomes, and that the ultimate "right" way to walk for the strongest body is to walk in all the ways natural for a human. I'd say that walking is the response of a muscle to the terrain you are walking over, the speed you're walking, what shoes you're wearing, and many other things. There is, for every situation, a natural way the environment is negotiated, but there is no single repetitive way for a human to move through every moment of every day.

Organisms can be studied at different levels, from proteins to cells to individuals to populations to ecosystems and to the universe. An ecologist typically investigates organisms in the context of a wide environment, while a biologist usually investigates at a more micro level. In the same way, a movement ecologist investigates movement in the context of the wider environment, while a biomechanist looks at movement in the microenvironment of the organism's own body.

My transition into thinking of movement relative to a natural context happened because of the internet. I went to college before the internet was a thing. It existed, but people didn't live in it the way they do now. Before then, the bulk of my human-to-human exchanges regarding movement happened in person, with people similar to me in background. My perspective on mechanics was constantly reinforced by the people who instructed me, and the people who were instructed by those same people.

In graduate school, I started coming up with questions beyond the curriculum offered there. I quickly found there were no academic papers on the models of movement I was considering. The biomechanics of pitching a baseball, wearing a pedometer 10,000 steps, and corrective exercise for knee pain, yes. The gait pattern of a single person on a treadmill compared to that individual's gait pattern walking over natural terrain with a group of fellow humans of varying ages, no.

After graduating and going forth to do the things this

biomechanist does, I became involved in many discussions with people outside of my bubble. People online who were not trained in biomechanics but who were expert movers, people with disabilities, other biomechanists who studied at different universities, people trained in anthropology, people who could and couldn't do a squat and were wondering why. I learned to watch my words and to strive for the most accurate written representation of my thoughts. I learned that not everyone holds the same definitions for things. With online dialogue, I was able to clarify some of the questions I began working on years ago in school. Through inspired insights, I refined my search, found better data, and realized that what I had learned was a minuscule fraction of what there was to know regarding biomechanics.

Alignment Matters was my second book—a publication comprising five years of blog posts discussing basic ideas surrounding movement form, how the visible body parts, like the head and shoulders and knees and hips, could and should be aligned with each other for various outcomes. In response to *Alignment Matters* and my first book (*Every Woman's Guide to Foot Pain Relief*), I spent years answering questions (online and in person), which typically required that I deepen my presentation to include the more complex model I had simplified for ease in writing. Eventually I started presenting, in layperson format, the more complex models, and my subsequent books offered more than "how to orient a body when still," such as how movement of the body works on a cellular level.

My book *Move Your DNA* explored these complex models, how our cells respond to movement, how changing the context of a movement changes its effect on our bodies. Despite the complexity of the content in *Move Your DNA*, there were still more layers to add, and in spending time answering questions about that book, I began presenting in my written pieces and correspondence an even more complex model of movement—including the idea that the effects of movement are not only deep to the skin.

A few years ago I realized that the sedentarism I have been writing about for a decade wasn't only of the body, but of thoughts as well. I don't mean (only) that people have a hard time moving their thoughts to consider new information, but that "we are unmoving" is the unacknowledged assumption underlying some of the most prevalent problems we are dealing with in areas of public health and safety, environmental science, and social issues. As I began to offer movement solutions for seemingly mundane things like foot pain and pelvic incontinence, many people responded, detailing why, for them, these movement solutions just weren't possible. Their inability to fit foot and hip exercises into their day was the result of the larger immobility *of their situation*. School, or work, or relationships, or work distribution within the home, was preventing their body parts from moving. They were immobilized by the expectations of a society, of their culture.

I believe the expansion to an ecological model in human body science—considering society's impact when we investigate human movement—is necessary for scientific clarity. In the same way a wildlife biologist cannot fully detail the natural behavior of wolves by studying 1,000 or even 100,000 wolves living independently in a zoo, the data gleaned from studying the way a human who has lived their life almost entirely inside, barely moving, moves their body on a treadmill in a laboratory is not necessarily what you want to use as the basis for all your foundational assumptions regarding human movement. As a biomechanist trying to understand how a body moves relative to the world, I have come to realize that an ecological model is the broadest, most accurate application of the physical laws of the universe to the human body. To continue to use a smaller model would be to not do my best work as a biomechanist.

At this point I am unable to accurately answer questions about human biomechanics—*how should I walk, how should I stand, how can I carry my baby more,* etc.—without a broader context. The questions I receive usually come with a fact gleaned from a study or book detailing "human movement"—the subjects of these studies being college-aged kinesiology students of Western European descent (which constitutes the bulk of biomechanical data). My answers typically begin with an explanation of assumptions, and measured populations, and reduction—things that many of the question-askers hadn't considered. For many, the publication of a research article in a peer-reviewed journal was the equivalent of truth (read "Proof" on page 26) and not a single data point in a much larger library of information. It's not that you have to take everything with a grain of salt so much as you must understand that this is what you have: a single grain of information.

In "What Is a Disease?" by Jackie Leach Scully (a paper I

recommend everyone read), Scully writes: "But science does not stand above the culture in which it operates, and the influences flow both ways."[1]

So, what are the influences of a sedentary culture on science, and how do the findings of research set up by a sedentary culture keep us sedentary? This is what I'm currently interested in understanding. I am working to flesh out how a sedentary culture develops and how that sedentary behavior permeates not only movement, but how we think of movement, how we research movement, how we create and use guidelines based on the conclusions of the aforementioned research, and how those guidelines promote further sedentary behavior.

That movement matters isn't earth-shattering news. It's pretty basic physiology, actually. But just as basic, although it takes a bit of explanation to get there, is that our lack of movement doesn't only affect our bodies negatively; it also negatively impacts the planet we live on.

I once heard humanitarian Ashley Judd say that it was abusive to point out a problem without offering a solution, and so as much as I feel this problem needs to be extremely well defined and thoroughly explained, alongside I'd like to suggest, at least in part, a solution: you need to move more than you do right now. You not only need to move more, you must also move better. You not only need to move more and better, you must also move with other people, and move through, around, and over some natural terrain. If you can't convince your tribe to move more, you must create a new tribe. Which often requires (ironically) that you move. Move at your job, or move jobs, move homes, or at least move furniture around or out of your home. Your contribution toward a solution to many problems, whether they're related to illness or finances or loneliness or boredom or feeding the underfed or freeing the oppressed, can often be "move more." Small and large issues alike can feel overwhelming, but often this is a result of trying to solve problems without changing anything about the life that created them. And so, allow me to show you how to move, for a better body, a better life, and a better world.

Movement Matters is a collection of essays that I've written over the last five years, usually in response to something I've read or witnessed that helped me deepen my understanding of biological models, the role of movement in nature and survival, and sedentary cultures. I've also included some of the questions I'm most frequently asked, and some helpful commentary I received on the topics I've selected. These essays are intended to educate, inspire, and motivate you towards a movement-based lifestyle, a lifestyle that honors both the body in which you dwell and the body upon which you reside.

My hope with *Movement Matters* is that a more robust model and deeper investigation of movement result in a movement revolution fashioned organically out of many smaller individual restorations of the natural types and frequencies of movement.

---

1. Scully, Jackie Leach. 2004. "What Is a Disease?" *EMBO Reports* 5 (7): 650–653.

MOVEMENT: OUTSOURCED

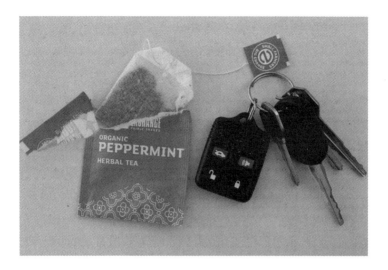

These items—an electronic car unlocker and a tea bag—are convenient. But what I've realized is, when we say or think "convenience," it's not as much about saving time as it is about reducing movement. We can grasp sedentary behavior as it relates to exercise because it's easy to see the difference between exercising one hour a day and not exercising one hour a day. My work, in the past, has been about challenging people to also be able to see the difference between exercising one hour a day and *not* exercising the other twenty-three. More subtle still—and what I'm asking you to do now—is to see how the choice to move is presented to you every moment of the day, but how most often we select the most sedentary choice without even realizing it.

Our daily life is composed of a lot of seemingly innocuous ways we've outsourced our body's work. One of the reasons I've begun focusing just as much on non-exercisey movements as I do on exercise-type movements is that I feel that the ten thousand outsourcings a day during the 23/24ths of your time hold the most potential for radical change. Be on the lookout for these things. To avoid the movements necessary to walk around to all the car doors, or just to avoid turning your wrist, or to avoid gathering your tea strainer and dumping the leaves and cleaning the strainer (in your dishwasher?), you have accepted a handful of garbage, plastic (future landfill), and a battery. To avoid the simplest movements, you have—without realizing it—required other humans somewhere else in the world to labor endlessly, destroy ecosystems, and wage war…for your convenience.

Sedentarism is very much linked to consumerism, materialism, colonialism, and the destruction of the planet. If you're not moving, someone else is moving for you, either directly, or indirectly by making STUFF to make not moving easier on you. You were born into a sedentary culture, so 99.9 percent of your sedentary behaviors are flying under your radar. Start paying attention. What do you see?

SCIENCE *moves*

Scientific ideas deserve close attention when and where they come up, but one must be alert to the whole of the scientific enterprise and anything even vaguely "scientific."

–JAMES E. MCCLELLAN III,
FROM *COLONIALISM & SCIENCE*

S cience is sometimes considered a set of facts rather than a process. Sedentary, unchanging, *unmoving* truths. But when you frequent academia and research, you'll find that science is in fact dynamic. Scientific models—the way problems are set up in order to investigate them—are simple to begin with, and as we learn from them, they become more complex. Often the answers that come from simple models are replaced with the answers that come from more complex models. This process repeats and repeats and repeats, and in every field of science the understanding has continued to expand or deepen, the "truths" moving in accordance with the model. If science is a pursuit, the work of a scientist is never-ending, for the movement of the model keeps science in motion.

MUSCLE: A SIMPLE MODEL

I use oversimplified models all the time. Sciences, like anatomy for example, typically require a step-by-step approach, where deeper understanding comes from studying additional layers. Once, in an article called "Have You Fallen for These Fitness Myths?"[2] I read that it was a myth that muscles lengthened, and that the Truth, according to their expert, was: "Muscles have what's called an origin and an insertion. Both are fixed and attached to bone. In order to lengthen it, you'd have to detach it and re-attach it farther down the bone."

First of all, muscles do get longer and shorter; this is how you're able to move. Your muscle's attachment points—often referred to as origin and insertion—are able to move away from each other without detachment and reattachment, thank goodness. We call

---

PART OF A WHOLE

We call a group of geese a flock and we call a group of sarcomeres a muscle. In school it's likely you were taught goose first and flock second, but when it comes to the body, we learn the groupings of parts first (i.e., a tissue type, like muscle). When you learn about muscle more deeply you'll find that, in the same way a flock moves only when each goose does, a muscle moves only when the sarcomeres that comprise it move. I could also say (and I am saying) that a goose flies because parts of it—like its wings and legs—move in a particular way, and similarly, a sarcomere only moves because its parts—the actin and myosin—do.

Note: A "gaggle of geese" refers specifically to a group of non-flying geese, a "skein" is group of flying geese, and a "flock" is just a group. You're welcome.

tissue that runs between attachment points "muscle," but really what we call muscle is long chains of units called sarcomeres, oriented in a way that allows them to move closer to or away from each other.

As you flex and extend a joint, each sarcomere on one side of the joint slides together and each on the other side slides apart, lengthening and shortening a muscle in that moment.

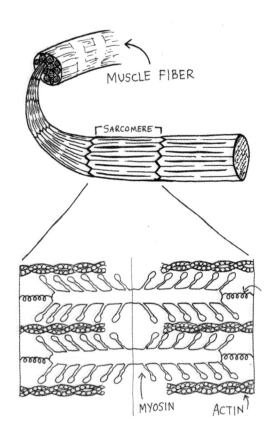

MUSCLE FIBER

SARCOMERE

MYOSIN   ACTIN

What I think the expert meant was, the amount a muscle can lengthen and shorten can't be changed (i.e., how much you can move is predetermined because the attachment points are set), as I'm assuming he knows that one of the basic properties of muscle is *extensibility*—the ability to move beyond its resting length. But even considering what I think he meant, the article still wasn't correct, as your body can change the number of sarcomeres between each attachment point and therefore the amount a muscle can lengthen and shorten.

When you assume the same position chronically or use your muscles in a limited and repetitive way, the mechanical environment senses, on the cellular level, where you spend the most time and adapts to make this static position easier (takes less energy) for your body. When repetitive positioning pushes a muscle's sarcomeres together with great frequency (i.e., shortens a muscle with great frequency), your body can respond by removing some sarcomeres so that the chain of them rests in a position that's ready for movement. Similarly, in muscles where each sarcomere is chronically positioned to a length where force generation is diminished, the body will add more sarcomeres so that the chain of them rests in a position that's ready for movement.

Your body and the movement it is capable of aren't as fixed as you've been led to believe. Yes, muscle attachment points are fixed, but the distance between them is not. Your muscles get longer or shorter as you use them, and in the greater picture, depending on how you use them.

I'm not sure what I found most frustrating about the article— that the information wasn't correct, that nobody seemed to do any fact-checking, or if it was, simply, that by implying it wasn't possible, this single news article may have discouraged thousands of people from lengthening and shortening their muscles while moving.

---

2. Deardorff, Julie. 2011. "Muscling Past Myths." *Chicago Tribune*, September 28. <articles.chicagotribune.com/2011-09-28/health/sc-health-0928-fitness-myths-20110928_1_fitness-myths-muscle-cells>

EXPAND YOUR MUSCLE MODEL

When I was eight, my mom gave me a pop-up book called *The Human Body* by Jonathan Miller for Christmas. I still love it and use it for work thirty years later.

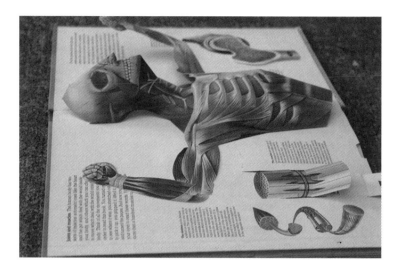

From the book: "When the ['move'] message arrives from the brain it releases a chemical which activates the muscles fibers and makes them slide into one another. By this means, the overall length of the muscle is shortened."

As you can imagine, we know more about muscle in 2016 than we did in 1984, and here's what I'd suggest adding to the updated version of *The Human Body*, if they updated pop-up books, which they don't: Sarcomeres don't only shorten lengthwise during contraction—they also bulge.

From the article "Where Do Muscles Get Their Power? Fifty-Year-Old Assumptions about Strength Muscled Aside":[3]

"One of the major discoveries that David Williams brought to light is that force is generated in multiple directions, not just along the long axis of muscle as everyone thinks, but also in the radial direction," said Thomas Daniel, UW professor of biology and co-author on the paper.

"This aspect of muscle force generation has flown under the radar for decades and is now becoming a critical feature of our understanding of normal and pathological aspects of muscle," Daniel added.

Historian Howard Zinn, in a speech discussing the selectively eliminated stories of human labor struggles, noted, "In graduate school, you get the same historical perspective as in elementary school, except with footnotes."

While I don't believe details are left out of muscular models to purposefully sway our thinking, I do think an introductory-level, narrow perspective can persist, even at advanced levels, when there's no robust system in place that notifies everyone when there are developments in scientific findings. Imagine how much more effective your certificate or college degree would be if it were like an iPhone, complete with a version number and mandatory updates in order to keep your knowledge software running smoothly and not slowing you down.

So, update! Adding the expanding (radial) motion of muscle to the shortening/lengthening movement of muscle explains how a contracting muscle moves the tissues both surrounding and embedded in that muscle—like blood vessels.

For decades—including when I was an undergraduate—blood flow to working muscles triggered at the onset of exercise (called exercise hyperaemia) was theorized to be caused by vasoactive substances signaling the arterioles inside the muscle to vasodilate (open up). However, there was no definitive support for involvement of any specific vasodilator. It was not until this last decade that mechanical triggers were explored:

> Given that the vessel wall is known to respond to mechanical stimuli such as shear stress...and cyclic stretch..., mechanical compression of the vasculature during contraction should be considered as a mechanism for exercise hyperaemia. Using ultrasound methods, it can be observed that the arteries of the human forearm are compressed and deformed during forceful contractions.[4]

Adding radial expansion of muscle to our movement model brings us a step closer to understanding how muscular contraction doesn't only result in a whole-body state of getting your person from point A to point B; your big movements are moving smaller parts within your person.

It's nice to see things come together. I mean expand.

You know what I mean.

---

3. ScienceDaily. 2013. "Where Do muscles Get Their Power? Fifty-Year-Old Assumptions About Strength Muscled Aside." July 12. <sciencedaily.com/releases/2013/07/130712102844.htm>

4. Clifford, P.S., Heidi A. Kluess, Jason J. Hamann, John B. Buckwalter and Jeffrey L. Jasperse. 2006. "Mechanical Compression Elicits Vasodilatation in Rat Skeletal Muscle Feed Arteries." *J Physiol* 572.2: 561–567.

Additional Sources

Williams, C. D., M. K. Salcedo, T. C. Irving, M. Regnier, T. L. Daniel. 2013. "The length-tension curve in muscle depends on lattice spacing." *Proceedings of the Royal Society B: Biological Sciences* 280 (1766): 20130697. DOI: 10.1098/rspb.2013.0697

Clifford, P.S. 2007. "Skeletal muscle vasodilatation at the onset of exercise." *J Physiol* 583.3: 825–833.

YOU'RE MORE THAN (TWO OF) YOUR PARTS

I'm interested in birthing stuff, not just because I'm a hopeless pelvis geek, but because I'm human and concerned with the process that propagates our species.

I was reading an old *National Geographic* when I stumbled on this passage by Dian Fossey: "One of the basic steps in saving a threatened species is to learn more about it: its diet, its mating and reproductive processes, its range patterns, its social behavior."[5]

As a nation we spend a lot of time and money studying these categories in the human animal, but have yet to invest much in understanding or quantifying what baseline values (e.g., nutrition, types of motion, type of community) are necessary for basic biological function. How can you figure out what's wrong if you haven't yet figured out what's right?

There are many ideas about women and birth handed down through the academic process, one of them being the "obstetrical dilemma." The obstetrical dilemma attempts to explain why human labor is so difficult (compared to that of other primates)—that if we had a wider pelvis it would be easier for the baby to come out, but if our pelvis were wider it would take more energy to walk, and so the tradeoff for being bipedal is difficult labors.

A few years ago I read an article titled "URI Anthropologist's Research Refutes Long-Held Theory on Human Gestation":[6]

"All these fascinating phenomena in human evolution—bipedalism, difficult childbirth, wide female hips, big brains, relatively helpless babies—have traditionally been tied together with the obstetric dilemma," said Holly Dunsworth, an anthropologist at the University of Rhode

Island and lead author of the research. "It's been taught in anthropology courses for decades, but when I looked for hard evidence that it's actually true, I struck out."

Recently ScienceDaily released the article "Evolution of Childbirth: Wider Hips Don't Make Locomotion Easier, so Why is Labor so Hard?"[7] The headline reads like breaking news, but not only was it written three years after Dunsworth's research, there have been many other studies showing that a "female" pelvis (typically wider than a man's) doesn't translate to a less efficient gait pattern.

> "The bottom line is that people with wider hips don't have higher costs for locomotion," [Daniel] Lieberman added. "In fact, if you look at old studies that compared how efficient men and women are, they have always showed no difference. We have long had plenty of data to disprove the idea that men are more efficient than women at walking and running—but now we know why it's wrong."

So what was wrong with the original model? Imagine tying a ten-pound weight to the end of a broom. The closer you hold the weight to the center of your body, the easier it is to hold; the farther away the weight, the harder it is to hold.

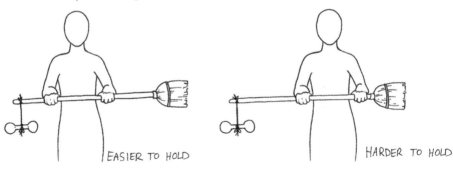

EASIER TO HOLD   HARDER TO HOLD

A similar leverage model was used to calculate which made more work for the lateral hip muscles: carrying a narrow or a wide pelvis. When you lift your leg to take a step, you remove the support from one side of the pelvis. In response, the lateral hip muscles contract (shorten) to hold the pelvis level as gravity tries to pull the unsupported side of the pelvis toward the ground.

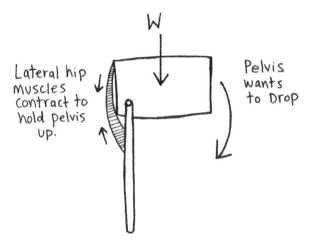

As in the broom model, a wider pelvis moves the weight farther from the axis of rotation at the hip, creating more work for the lateral hip.

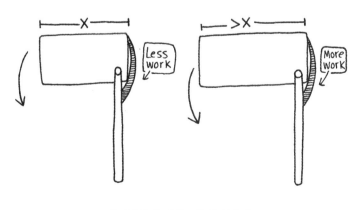

The physics in the original model was correct, but it wasn't the most accurate model to use.

Mathematical models in biology are tough—you always have to simplify. In the case of the assumption that women are less efficient walkers than men, the model used to determine *whole-body efficiency of a gender of a species* included two parts—the pelvis and a femur. As you can imagine, calculating whole-body, whole-gender, whole-species information from two parts of a trillion-part body has limitations.

The newer model was improved by including more of the anatomy that assists in supporting the pelvis (i.e., adding more parts). By creating a *five*-part model—adding the shank, ankle, and foot (which, P.S., is really at least thirty-three parts in itself, but is represented here by a solid one) and the muscles that connect them to the pelvis—scientists found out why a wide pelvis doesn't reduce gait efficiency. In short, when you have wide hips (or narrow ones, for that matter), you don't ONLY have wide hips; your other parts are shaped to normalize forces between shapes. Sizes of the femoral head and neck might be larger or longer, tendons can be different lengths, etc. Said another way, you can't tell much by looking at a small area or a couple of parts of the body. As we've seen demonstrated here, conclusions based on simplified models can be misleading.

This also goes for determining generalizations about function by looking at parts. A pile of pelves or femurs from a bunch of different people tells you very little; you must see the entire structure (and I don't mean the entire skeleton, but the entire *body*) for accurate data collection.

Almost everything you and I have been told about the body is based on a simple model. You and your parts—your organs, knees, breasts, balls, and biome (I went for the alliteration)—don't exist in a vacuum. You're a trillion-part meatball, responding to the ideas in your head, the food in your fridge, the air in your lungs, the people in your day planner, the orientation of your body, and the number of emails in your inbox. Let us work on the more difficult (math) problems, not always begin our research with the assumption that the difficulties experienced by a sedentary culture are the same difficulties experienced by all *Homo sapiens* throughout time, and start funding studies that help determine our baseline. Let's do Dian Fossey proud.

---

5. Fossey, Dian. 1970. "Making Friends with Mountain Gorillas." *National Geographic* 137(1): 48–67.

6. University of Rhode Island. 2012. "URI Anthropologist's Research Refutes Long-Held Theory on Human Gestation." Press Release. August 27. <uri.edu/news/releases/?id=6358>

7. ScienceDaily. 2013. "Evolution of Childbirth: Wider Hips Don't Make Locomotion Easier, so Why Is Labor so Hard?" March 13. <sciencedaily.com/releases/2015/03/150313094557.htm>

Additional Sources

Warrener, Anna G., Kristi L. Lewton, Herman Pontzer, Daniel E. Lieberman. 2015. "A Wider Pelvis Does Not Increase Locomotor Cost in Humans, with Implications for the Evolution of Childbirth." *PLOS ONE* 10(3): e0118903.

PROOF

We are a society obsessed with proof. As a presenter of non-mainstream information for the general public, I often get requests like "show me the proof that trampolines are good or bad." The following evolved from my response to a gentlemen wanting proof a "treadmill was useless." (Not my words, nor my original article's meaning either—the original article explores "Junk Food Walking," and describes some of the physiological differences between overground and treadmill walking.)

The thing is, I can't explain why running on a treadmill is "no good." I don't believe running on a treadmill is no good, only that it is not equivalent to overground walking. When I write, as I have written many times on the difference between overground and treadmill walking, I don't write about how they're similar—that you can get your heart rate up the same or burn the same calories. Instead, I consider how they're different—specifically their biomechanical differences.

I don't write to make anyone feel good or bad, I just tend to write about ideas that are not held by many. I often get requests for "research" or "proof" for these new ideas, and many are looking for a single study that reads like a headline, as in "Treadmill Walking Causes Knee Osteoarthritis." I don't have any of those. What I do have are lots of articles, from different journals, in different fields, each with a different piece of a puzzle.

Research titles *shouldn't* read like magazine headlines; every study presents just a tiny aspect of something. Scientists look at thousands of articles to get an idea of how something works. A conclusion drawn from a single research paper might change when compared to one drawn from a more robust literature review.

For example, I think of the hundreds of published articles on pelvic floor science that support the use of pelvic floor contraction as a means of improving pelvic floor function. When you run an evidence-based practice, getting articles like this are helpful because they support the therapies you offer. But what happens when newer data comes out showing that surface EMG[8] or manual vaginal readings[9] aren't necessarily a valid measure in determining an improvement in function? There isn't a research database manager that goes back and flags all previous pelvic floor studies using these methods with a "Sorry! This study is no longer valid as a portion of the methods has been shown to misconstrue conclusions." This is why a wide literature view will give you the best shot at gathering the clearest picture and why a single article will not suffice.

My assumption is that if you're interested in evidence, you're interested in all of it. And that if you use a scientific publication to support your behavior, you are extensively reviewing the literature yourself, and that a new idea sparks a surge in research and reading, and not only in online commenting.

Proof is tricky. By searching Google Scholar or PubMed using key phrases such as "comparing overground and treadmill running biomechanics," you will find not only articles comparing the two, but also the history of assumptions. You can read that before the 1970s, physiologists created a simple model that set them as equal (sort of like you can call apples and oranges equal if you refer to each as a fruit), to justify using a treadmill as an easy means of gathering data about movement.

It was only in 1972 that someone with training in physics thought it was quite possible they were different, and tested them.

> A question arises, however, as to whether the results from treadmill studies can be directly applied to running overground. Personal conversations with three internationally recognized physiologists...indicated that such an application is valid on the basis of fundamental mechanics. That is, in a system involving movement of a man relative to a surface, it makes no difference whether he moves over the ground or the ground (treadmill belt) moves beneath him. The researchers agree that except for air resistance it can be assumed there is no difference in running on the two types of surfaces....Even less interest has been shown in the biomechanical aspects of this comparison. Consequently, the authors were unable to locate even one study in the literature dealing with the biomechanics of running under these different conditions. Since results derived from treadmill studies will continue to be applied to performance on stationary surfaces, it is essential that comparative investigations be made to determine the validity of this procedure.[10]

The conclusion of this paper stated that "the biomechanics of treadmill running differ significantly from those associated with overground running."

For me, the research process goes something like this: I think, "Treadmill and overground movement look similar, but are they different?" I go look up "overground walking and treadmill walking," and read all those papers. From these papers I might create a list of how they're different—maybe the muscles used are different or the joints are moving at different angles or rates (e.g., treadmill walking uses more hip flexion). Then I look up different musculoskeletal ailments and see that excessive hip flexion is a risk factor for ailments X and Y. Then I think back to the biomechanics research (or gait textbooks or literature reviews) I've already read about tissue adaptation to repetitive use, and then I think back to a physics class and consider the belt of a treadmill and how you have to move over it, and then back to an anatomy class and recall which muscles worked in which way, and it takes a long time and I should really get a hobby.

I would never say treadmills are worse than not moving at all, or that "exercise machines have no benefits," yet I will say that there are differences between them, and how they're different can be a risk factor for certain musculoskeletal ailments, because I think you should know. Their being the same has been implied to you for so long (without proof, I might add) that hearing they're *not* the same can feel threatening, and you need proof that your behavior (treadmill walking, in this case) can harm you before you do the work to change your habit.

I popped open the book *Ill Nature* by Joy Williams last night (I often pop open a book to the middle and read a few pages as I believe that will deliver some sort of message) and this is what it said:

> Though it's quite apparent that the environment has been grossly polluted and the natural world abused and defiled, you seem to prefer to continue pondering effects rather than preventing causes. You want proof, you insist on proof. A Dr. Lave from Carnegie-Mellon—and he's an expert, an economist and an environmental expert—says that scientists will

> have to prove to you that you will suffer if you don't
> become less of a "throw-away society."...To try to
> appease your appetite for proof, for example, scien-
> tists have been leasing for experimentation forty-six
> pristine lakes in Canada....They've been intention-
> ally contaminating many of the lakes with a variety
> of pollutants...[in] one of the *boldest experiments in*
> *lake ecology ever conducted.* They've been doing
> this since 1976! And what they've found so far is that
> pollutants are really destructive. It took about eight
> years to make this happen...and it will take hundreds
> of years for the lakes to recover. They think.

I think many people believe science approves or disapproves of a behavior. To get proof is to ensure you've made the right decision, and lately I've been wondering if we've mistaken science for proof.

Though words like *law* are often used to describe equations used in science, this does not imply that the derivatives of science are infallible. Proofs (i.e., absolutes) exist in math and in logic. In science there is only evidence to support a theory—making science provisional. The best or most widely accepted theory is only the best explanation among all available alternatives.

If you're looking for headlines in the evidence to help you know for sure that something in the modern world is hurting *your body*, it will be difficult to find. While researchers are perfectly happy destroying the environment to prove that it can be destroyed, we are not so liberal with people—anymore. We don't create and get approval for studies setting up a population to do something harmful to see how bad the outcomes are—the times when we have in the past are deplorable.

When striving for an evidence-based life, consider that your most relevant evidence is your body. If your body works and feels great, no worries; what you're doing is apparently working for you. If you're experiencing an issue, expand the evidence you've considered, keeping in mind you're not going to find a headline, but a rabbit hole.

Does something like walking on the ground instead of on a treadmill put you at enormous risk or cost you so greatly that you need a double-blind, randomized, placebo-controlled study (if you can figure out how this would be possible, call me) supporting a transition to overground walking before you'd consider doing it? Ask yourself why that is.

8. Auchincloss, C. C., and L. McLean. 2009. "The Reliability of Surface EMG Recorded from the Pelvic Floor Muscles." *Journal of Neuroscience Methods* 182(1): 85–96. <europepmc.org/abstract/MED/19539646/reload=0;jsessionid=zjn-B4xSCvtwlifHQMr4D.0>

9. Bø, Kari, and Hanne Borg Finckenhagen. 2008. "Vaginal Palpation of Pelvic Floor Muscle Strength: Inter-Test Reproducibility and Comparison Between Palpation and Vaginal Squeeze Pressure." *Acta Obstetricia et Gynecologica Scandinavica* 80(10): 883–887. <onlinelibrary.wiley.com/doi/10.1034/j.1600-0412.2001.801003.x/abstract?deniedAccessCustomised-Message=&userIsAuthenticated=false>

10. Nelson, R. C., C. J. Dillman, P. Lagasse, and P. Bickett. 1972. "Biomechanics of Overground Versus Treadmill Running." *Medicine and Science in Sports* 4(4): 233–240. <ncbi.nlm.nih.gov/pubmed/4648586>

PUTTING ALL YOUR EGGS IN ONE COMMENT BASKET

The other day I watched a YouTube video[11] featuring two children arguing over the weather. I felt compelled to share it because it reminded me of many online comment boards and discussions the world over.

"It's raining!" one says. "No, it's SPRINKLING," says the other. And back and forth they go, both citing their authority ("my mom," in both cases). Neither one of them sees that what they're saying is 99.9 percent the same thing—that it's wet outside, that water is falling from the sky, that they need a jacket, etc. Round and round they go, repeating the words given to them by someone else.

Then a tiny moderator steps in. "Let's just go outside!" she says. Collect some data and we can test it for ourselves! Let's get away from the comments section on a computer—I mean, this preschool—where nothing we're talking about is even occurring!

I was fresh from watching the clip when someone sent me the article: "Eggs Unlimited: An Extraordinary Tale of Scientific Discovery."[12] It's common knowledge that women are born with all the eggs they'll ever have (which means the cell that eventually became YOU once resided within your mom's ovaries when she was in *her* mother's womb; in other words, you-in-some-form were once in your grandmother).

Only it turns out that the you-were-once-in-your-granny-thing might not be correct for every egg (read: person): women might be able to produce egg cells throughout a lifetime.[13]

Ten years ago, when the scientist making this discovery started publishing stuff that challenged the dogma, the dialogue wasn't as friendly as you'd expect between human beings all interested in the same thing (i.e., understanding how human bodies work):

> When Tilly published his study in the journal *Nature* in 2004 the fertility community was not pleased. Understandably, he was subjected to rigorous scientific scrutiny that continued for many years afterwards, but some comments were designed to be deliberately cruel.
>
> "It was discouraging to hear so many people voice negative comments about the work, and many of the comments were not based on science but were personal opinions and beliefs," Tilly said.
>
> The work was carried out on mouse ovaries, the standard animal model, and some critics suggested the findings may be an artifact of murine tissue. One reviewer helpfully suggested that humans are not big mice, unless you live in Disneyland.[14]

(What I find ironic about the Disneyland comment is that all the original research from the 1950s—the "proof" that women come with all their eggs—used rats, monkeys, cows, and pigs. If you're going to criticize a study for something, you can't be relying on another study doing the very same thing.)

Anyhow, my point is, because science (all information, really) is constantly In Progress, the quick (and/or rude) dismissal of something new isn't really the most scientific course of action. Refusing to investigate new ideas, reexamine old ones, and hold space for progress all limits science. Being certain about "how things work" when your certainty is based on a limited perspective can leave many avenues unexplored. For example, if women *do* continuously make eggs, then what are other potential causes of menopause or infertility? If we've concluded that eggs are fixed in number, we'll never answer these questions because we're already heading down the wrong path when we set up our investigations.

So anyhow, the video of the kids debating the weather made me think. When someone writes or says something you don't believe, start by heading to your own sources. Review the information, old and new—become your own authority. Read *everything*. Collect your own data. Be kind. Go outside in the rain.

---

11. Find the great debate here: youtu.be/3sKdDyyanGk.

12. Connor, Steve. 2012. "Eggs Unlimited: An Extraordinary Tale of Scientific Discovery." *Independent,* April 6. <independent.co.uk/life-style/health-and-families/health-news/eggs-unlimited-an-extraordinary-tale-of-scientific-discovery-7624715.html>

13. Gura, Trisha. 2012. "Reproductive Biology: Fertile Mind." *Nature,* November 14. <nature.com/news/reproductive-biology-fertile-mind-1.11805>

14. Connor, Steve. (See note 12.)

DON'T BE A STUPID

In *Huffington Post* article "Sitting May Harm Health Says AARP,"
Ann Brenoff discusses the metaphor likening sitting habits to
smoking habits. She isn't all that impressed by the information and
isn't going to stop sitting because, frankly, it appears she believes that
"mounting evidence" deserves sarcastic quotes.

> Why don't I stand, you ask? For a few reasons. I once
> worked next to a woman who insisted on placing her
> office computer on a pedestal so that she could stand
> all day in front of it instead of sitting. For her, it worked
> out well. For everyone else, not so much.
>
> For one thing, nobody appreciated being towered over.
> Her standing blocked our already limited view of office
> life (mostly people sitting in front of their computers
> in little cubicles) and projected her already-loud voice
> to an intrusive level. An office community is a delicate
> balance of personal needs and consideration of others.
> The others must trump the personal needs if there is to
> be harmony and productivity.
>
> It took mere minutes before my co-worker's standing
> raised people's blood pressure. She eventually sat down.

I get it. She doesn't want to stand because she feels that standing
disrupts others' personal needs and so forth. To each their own—or
to each everyone else's own, I guess.

But look at this part (emphasis mine): "You may never convince
me that sitting is the greatest threat to my health; whereas smoking
certainly remains one of the chart toppers. **Smoking is a choice
that some stupid people make...**"

I read this as saying that people who smoke do so because they are stupid, and people who sit do so because they are considerate.

This attitude, that those who are doing the "right" thing are somehow smarter or better than those who aren't, doesn't appear to contribute to our health or happiness.

I guarantee that no matter how informed or well-read or degreed or dressed up or dressed down or organicked (a word, right?) or McDonalded or well-behaved or radical-ed up your life is, there is someone out there, right now, *who is doing it better than you*. There is someone out there messing up their kids less, eating better, doing more for the planet, doing more for humankind, using less fuel, giving more money, and being kinder to others. Which, by the reasoning used in the quoted article, makes YOU the stupid one.

People who do not share your views or behaviors are not stupid; they just don't share your views. They may never share your views, in the exact same way that you may never share theirs. Who's to say which views are correct?

Your faith in your beliefs is equal in magnitude to the faith of every other person on this planet in their own beliefs. Every second of time you spend lamenting that others don't think like you is time spent not honoring your beliefs. If you believe improvements in your personal health, the environment, and to human rights are that great, wouldn't your time be better spent actually working on them?

Before you so easily drop the "S" bomb on others, realize that someone has just dropped the Stupid all over your head. And it sucks to be stupided on. The end.

P.S. This is a letter I am writing to myself; I'm just letting you look at it.

SOMETIMES SCIENCE IS SEDENTARY

Biomechanics is the study of mechanical laws relating to the movement or structure of a living organism. But applying mechanical laws to living things is tricky, because the tissues that comprise the body aren't as easy to model as metals are. For example, I might want to figure out how much work it is for a bicep to curl up a thirty-pound weight. And so I make my diagram, setting the upper and lower arm bones as levers (i.e., rigid). "Rigid" is a key term here, because it's another way of saying the arm bones don't bend themselves, even though they do. We're taught how not to consider all the movement when we build a model because, well, it's easier that way. So I guess this is really an important piece to consider here—not only are the number of moving parts reduced to a few, but the parts that do remain are set to "still" before a solution is calculated.

I'm aware of the sedentary nature of biomechanics problems because biomechanics is my field and this is how it's done. It blew me away, though, when I learned of a similar phenomenon in cellular biology. Only this time it wasn't the model that was rendered static—it was the subject of investigation.

It turns out that all studies on cellular movement have occurred in the classic cell-culture petri dish, allowing only for 2-D movement. Captive, immobilized, sedentary cells serve as the foundation for our understanding of cellular biology. Upon investigating cellular movement for the first time in 3-D matrix (which is the natural habitat for your body's cells), the researchers "discovered" a new movement—meaning that after studying cells and drawing conclusions from those observations for decades, they finally observed a cell's natural movement (within an unnatural or artificial 3-D environment).

> "We think it's a very important normal physiological mechanism of cell movement that has not been characterized previously," [Ryan] Petrie said....
>
> "When a cell is in the matrix, the nucleus tends to be at the back of the cell, and the cell body is very tubular in shape," Petrie said. "It really looked like a piston."
>
> They found that the nucleus is actually pulled forward by the actin filaments that connect the nucleus to the front of the cell. This movement "pressurizes" the cell. The scientists were also able to identify the protein components responsible for moving the nuclear piston, including actomyosin, vimentin and nesprin.
>
> "The pressure itself is what pushes the plasma membrane," Petrie said.
>
> Because this only happened to cells moving in the three-dimensional cell-created matrix and not cells moving in other substrates, the researchers note that the cells must be sensing their physical environment to determine what type of movement to use.[15]

As I've said before, studying biological organisms in a movement-limited environment leads to conclusions that do not apply to that same organism in its natural and movement-rich habitat. This goes for orcas, humans—and individual cells, as researchers have just "discovered."

In light of a progression towards "evidence-based" living, what happens now? Should all previous studies done in captivity be labeled as such? Should we, personally, flag everything we think we know about cells and biology with "needs adjustment"?

One step I take is to always assume that whatever model I'm working with, whatever data I have in hand, is likely incredibly tiny in scope compared to the universe in which we are conducting our science. The data we have on cells is absolutely correct in the context of the 2-D environment it's been performed in; the work to be done now is to recognize the 2-D nature of our perspective…on everything. We have never arrived at an answer; there is always further to go. When science is sedentary, it's no longer science. Like us, it needs movement to survive.

---

15. PennNews. 2014. "Penn-NIH Team Discovers New Type of Cell Movement in 3D Matrix." Press release. August 28. <news.upenn.edu/news/penn-nih-team-discover-new-type-cell-movement-3d-matrix>

DEAR KATY

Q   WOULD YOU EVER WALK ON A TREADMILL?

A   If a treadmill were my only option for moving, I certainly would. Just last week I flew to a large city to attend a funeral, and the travel, plus the lack of any outdoor space to walk through and a few other extenuating circumstances, made the hotel treadmill the best option for me that day. I'm not against treadmills, I'm just for understanding the difference between treadmill and over-ground walking.

Q   REALISTICALLY, WHAT AMOUNT OF RESEARCH DO I NEED TO READ TO STAY INFORMED? HOW MUCH DO YOU READ?

A   I don't think "informed" is a whole-body state, although I do think you can specialize in a fraction of a single topic by studying it for a long period of time. Being informed includes knowing that subject's history—all of the hypotheses currently being considered as well as those discarded along the way, and why. To maintain an updated position (as if it were possible to keep truly up to date on the ever-expanding body of scientific data) I read ten to twenty articles per week. I don't have a rule to read ten to twenty; the articles I read are driven by the thoughts that I think and the questions that I formulate. I'm a very curious person, and those curiosities lead me, daily, down the path outlined in "Proof." I'm also extremely fortunate to have thousands of people who know the questions I'm interested in understanding and send me articles daily.

In response to their gracious contribution of interest and eyeballs, I try to convert their gifts into small paragraphs and shared links I believe they might be interested in, creating a cycle of service and generosity of knowledge that I'm grateful to be a part of.

Q WHAT PERCENTAGE OF YOUR LIFE'S DECISIONS ARE EVIDENCE-BASED?

A Given that there's hardly research on anything (given all the possible questions to ask) I'd say less than 10 percent, although I'm totally making up that number because I've never taken hard data regarding my every choice. I have read many textbooks and thousands of research articles, but these are focused on a narrow topic. When I need to make a choice on something, if I think there might be research on it, I'll investigate it as best I can, trying to think out of the box, giving attention to the merits of the currently accepted hypothesis but also criticisms of it. I think of science as always moving forward, but not always straight ahead. Even a cursory glance at the history of how many facts we all hold dear—that vitamins exist, for example, and that specific diseases erupt when we're without them—shows that there were scientific debates over these facts for hundreds of years (and let me tell you, people got nasty. As in, internet comments section nasty). Science is dynamic and it's only hindsight that reveals if the hypothesis you were using for a decision was slightly to the right or left of where science ended up on the matter, which is okay. Certainty doesn't bring me comfort so much as assuming responsibility both for the decision and outcome does.

NATURE *moves*

Amid all the revolutions of the globe, the economy of Nature has been uniform...and her laws are the only things that have resisted the general movement. The rivers and the rocks, the seas and the continents, have been changed in all their parts; but the laws which direct those changes, and the rules to which they are subject, have remained invariably the same.

—JOHN PLAYFAIR

The word "nature" and its definition are, obviously, created and used by humans. Nature is regularly defined as both *all* that is in the physical universe as well as how the universe works—with the exception of humans. The online Oxford dictionary defines nature as: "The phenomena of the physical world collectively, including plants, animals, the landscape, and other features and products of the earth, as opposed to humans or human creations." Once again, we're defining nature as *all* that is in the physical universe, as well as how the universe works—with the exception of humans. We might also use a more local definition of nature to describe a particular environment that includes all the phenomena of the collective world and all the products of the earth—except for humans or things humans have created. Wilderness is a further classification of nature, meaning a place untrammeled—not significantly altered or impacted—by human activities and home only to wild animals, not humans.

However you use these terms, it's important to be aware that at their most basic level, they imply or state outright that humans are not a part of the rest of the world and/or are very different from all other things.

Here are my thoughts on the matter. Ponderings on "human nature" and also on humans *in* nature likely came about once we were no longer living in what we now call nature or wilderness. Once the walls of our dwellings served as a physical barricade between nature and us, we needed language naming *that of which we were no longer a part*. Words that defined our separateness allowed us to speak clearly about our separateness, and thus we weren't only separated physically, but also in our minds. Our perception, shaped both by the way we use our body and by the way we use words, is that we fall outside of the natural world and its laws.

Science cannot be done outside the culture doing it, and so I propose that our belief in our separatism is an unconscious yet pervasive assumption in our scientific exploration into how the human animal works—and that it has somewhat limited our progress in certain fields of study. Which isn't to imply that science is necessarily wrong because of this, but that the questions and answers that comprise science are created by the minds doing the asking and answering, and that these question-asking minds are shaped by their personal experience.

If investigations into the inner workings of the human body, of illness of the body, of the solutions to illnesses, are being executed by minds perceiving that humans are not subject to the same laws as all other things in the universe, then the gathering and integrating of data on "how humans work" is to some degree limited. How does one accurately model a human that is, by our own definition of nature, not a part of any natural system?

The scientific process requires a series of reductions and the isolation of variables, and these are typically noted as they're being done. What hasn't been thoroughly documented in each case is the often underlying, not-stated, and likely not even perceived assumption that we think of humans as *the sole unique thing in the universe.*

We are currently living in a culture that separates us from what we define and label as nature, and we seem to be suffering the physical and mental effects of this separation. Yet because we do not see ourselves as belonging to the animal kingdom—as needing clean water and air and food and movement, just as all other wild animals do—our research begins by framing the symptoms of being in captivity as the problem. (We see this in many other captive animals, and I describe it in detail in *Move Your DNA*: cardiovascular disease, musculoskeletal ailments, diabetes, anxiety, depression, and many other modern health problems can be traced to our lack of movement, and our lack of movement in nature.) The research striving to heal us is informed by a worldview that sees us as essentially separated from the "natural" world—which one could argue is our problem in the first place. How can science offer solutions

EVERYTHING IS NATURE, BUT...

I assert that everything is nature, so when I say in this book that humans are living outside of nature, I sound like I'm contradicting myself. When we say that humans live outside of nature, what's really happening is that unlike human animals in the past, many humans are living in a way that requires them to consume natural resources at an unprecedented (arguably unnatural) rate. These humans and everything they make still operate within a natural ecosystem and are subject to natural law, but they differ in behavior from other animals in that they are heavily buffered, physically, by human-made materials and technologies for life-support purposes.

This all being stated, repeatedly writing that many humans are still in nature but thoroughly buffered from wilderness gets tedious, so for many essays I'll often refer to "humans in nature" in the commonly understood sense (i.e., regularly exposed to the wilderness without the numerous buffers developed in the last few hundred years); ditto for "humans out of nature" (i.e., those thoroughly buffered).

Also, that everything is nature makes it difficult to debate any lifestyle as unnatural, which is why I tend to question the sustainability of our choices rather than the naturalness of them.

to our health, economic, and cultural crises if no one thinks to set up questions investigating what some increasingly recognize as the fundamental issue: We cannot flourish away from this vast and wild thing we have labeled nature?

ANALOGOUS

Nature—especially trees and rivers—has been a great influence on how I think about movement. Through studying how trees and rivers are shaped, I learned the role physical forces play not only in their formation, but also in the form—the shape—we observe when we're out hiking in the wilderness.

When I look at trees, I see branches that have grown in a particular geometry—in terms of their number, thickness, and direction—to best optimize the sunlight, their ability to grab carbon from the air (to make their mass), and withstand the loads (bends, created by the wind) of their home without breaking. All of these inputs, plus their genes, create their shape. Blood vessels operate similarly; they branch opportunistically, and change their diameters and numbers (capillaries) based on their environment—that is, the forces placed upon them, created by your lifestyle and habitat. Your blood vessels are always monitoring their environment and responding, by adapting their shape to best survive in the environment in which you've placed them.

To stand alongside a river is to stand alongside a blood vessel of the earth, and from watching it you can get a sense of what's happening inside of you, especially if you are lucky enough to visit the river often and observe how its shape changes over time. The things that steer (affect the fluid dynamics of) a river's flow—changes to the speed and direction of flow due to branching, the temperature, the "pressure" of the system—are the same things that affect the fluid dynamics of your arterial and venous system. The pressure of a river will grow new "capillaries" (as do you) to deal with new volumes flowing through a particular area; when you block an artery, or river, it can create collateral flow to deal with the situation, and a rushing river will slowly carve away at its own sides.

Watching a river over a month will give you insights into how your internal rivers perform over an hour. Watching a river over a year will give you insights into how your internal rivers behave over a day. Watching a river over a millennium will give you insights into how your internal rivers change over your lifetime. The mechanics of the natural, living world are the same whether you're talking rivers, trees, humans, tigers, or cells; the only thing that varies is the scale. If you could see yourself as clearly as you see the river, what ails you would be less mysterious, less confusing. Taking action to change your course would become easier.

THIGMOMORPHOGENESIS[1]

I don't mind signs. I mind signs that don't communicate what the sign placer actually means. Writing "Tree climbing is unsafe" when

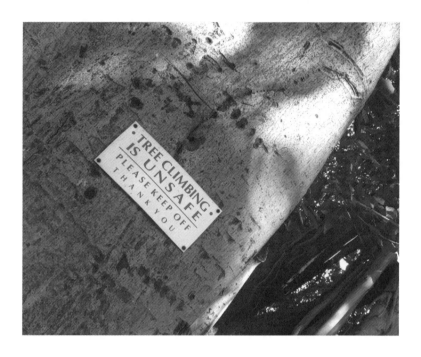

you mean "Please stay off the trees because we don't have money to pay for the injuries of inexperienced climbers" or "This is a nature reserve/park and the human-to-tree interaction is higher than it would be in nature—please climb trees in the wilderness or on your property" is lazy. Implying that climbing is dangerous is lazy. Perhaps it's also an indication that we don't see interactions between trees and humans as beneficial to either party and that while we recognize wind, water, fire, birds, bugs, bears, and a bunch of other animals as a tree's natural associates, human animals don't put themselves on the list of loads natural to trees. This despite the tons of food humans have obtained from trees for eons—obtained, of course, via climbing the trees.

I get that many humans behave thoughtlessly, but I also think it's possible that part of our thoughtless behavior is due to not spending more time in trees, and being told that nature is dangerous. What if we posted signs stating, "Your body is too weak and unskilled to move through nature safely" and "Forests were cut down so you could live in more comfort and do less movement, and therefore your body has become weak and there are hardly any trees left, so it's best to not climb these"? Why not post the facts instead of "Tree climbing is unsafe"?

---

1. The process by which plants alter their growth patterns via mechanical sensation (wind, rain, animal interactions).

SIGN WHAT YOU MEAN

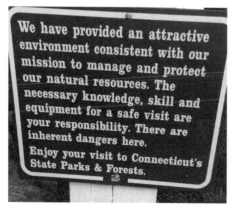

There are a lot of words on this sign, but it does a good job of explaining the issue and noting where the responsibility of personal safety truly lies: with you.

Photo credit: Johanna Lamb

SHAPED BY THE TREES

Numerous times throughout my formal education I have been taught the anatomy and capabilities of "human" ankles, e.g., normal maximum adult dorsiflexion—pulling toes toward the shin—is seventeen degrees.[2] And then, boom, someone studied the ankles of another group of modern humans, the Twa—Ugandan hunter-gatherers—who climb trees for the food they need, and found these humans' normal range of dorsiflexion to be greater than forty-five degrees.[3]

The ankle bones of the Twa are shaped like ours are, but their muscles have a different shape because they use their bodies differently than we do. They climb, and thus their bodies have adapted to climbing by growing muscles that allow for greater range of ankle motion.

Most of what I have been taught about how "human ankles" work is really how the ankles of people who don't use their ankles very much work. Which is fine, but not only did my textbooks (often titled some variation on "Human Anatomy and Physiology," suggesting they were definitive and comprehensive) and professors of my human anatomy courses fail to include even a cursory note on the matter, I don't think it had ever been pointed out to them.

Further, the biology, psychology, and sociology classes I took based *their* content on the assumption that the human brain became intellectually superior to other animals' because the modern human body was *clearly* unsuited for tree climbing. The explanation that the modern shape of our huge brain is relative to a modern ankle shape that renders us unable to climb trees fails to acknowledge that our ankles are tight because we don't, in fact, climb trees. What makes us different from other human animals and non-human animals on the planet is not our capacity for movement, but the movements we actually perform.

We've shaped an entire science to make sense of *our* culture's lack of particular movements. And what's even more impactful on how we move in the future is that we've defined our capabilities brought about by this lack of movement as an inherent property of our entire species.

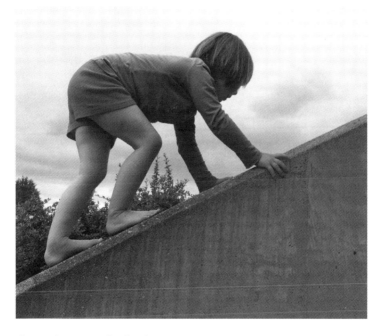

If you check the CDC reference at the end of this essay, you'll see twenty-five degrees of ankle dorsiflexion for a three-year-old girl is normal in our culture. This three-year old, however, who's never worn conventional heeled (calf-muscle-shortening) foot-wear, has been walking miles and miles with her family tribe, has grown up without chairs and couches (we squat and floor-sit at home), and climbs everything, often, is exhibiting her Twa-like ankle range of motion in this picture.

2. Centers for Disease Control and Prevention. 2010. "Normal Joint Range of Motion Study." Nov. 29. <cdc.gov/ncbddd/jointrom> Referring to study: Soucie, J.M., C. Wang, A. Forsyth, S. Funk, M. Denny, K.E. Roach, D. Boone, and the Hemophilia Treatment Center Network. 2010. "Range of Motion Measurements: Reference Values and a Database for Comparison Studies." *Haemophilia*, November 11.

3. Venkataraman, Vivek V., Thomas S. Kraft, and Nathaniel J. Dominy. 2013. "Tree Climbing and Human Evolution." *Proceedings of the National Academy of Sciences of the United States of America* 110(4): 1237–1242.

FIRST HIKE

From birth, my kids were always carried on walks, and from the time they could walk, we allowed them to go the distance at their own (slow) pace. I remember my son's first "real" hike. I say "real" because the first hundred walks felt like herding cats. The wide, groomed pathways we initially gravitated toward (free of debris, easy to walk on) gave him space to stagger in circles until he was tired and ready to go home. Or maybe that was just me.

On his "first real hike" we opted to go off the paved path near our home and down to the dirt trail slightly below instead. The next hour was pure magic. This kid, now facilitated by nature's walls, was focused on the narrow walkway ahead and proceeded to run/walk for over a mile, stopping only to fall, inspect some grass, poke a slug, and smell the flowers.

I don't spend a lot of time writing about stuff I don't know—mostly because writing about what I do know is challenging enough, and why be masochistic about it—but something occurred to me on this walk.

Humans have walked, collectively, long distances throughout time. Walking is a reflex, meaning it comes naturally to humans. What makes it so hard, then, to get our children walking? Let's assume that the parent is modeling regular walking behavior; why don't more kids catch on and walk in a way that would help out their tribe, i.e., forward, and more efficiently?

I've read about the psychological phenomenon of offering a child too many options, overwhelming them with broad questions, such as "What do you want to eat?" when they are surveying the crammed aisles in the grocery store. Perhaps having too many options is not a "natural" phenomenon in itself and renders a child unable to decide. Much better, say the experts, to offer them a choice, as in "Would you like eggs or cereal?" or "The red tights or the green shorts?"

Why not do the same thing with a trail: "Do you want to go back the way we came, or forward along this narrow path?"

It became clear to me that the size of the path was an important variable in the way that my son walked. The easier the path (wide, flat, debris-free), the lesser the challenge, and the lesser the challenge, the less interest he had in walking. He wasn't tired; he was bored. Adults can stay the course on wide, groomed pathways, but perhaps that's because we're aware of the health benefits of what we're doing.

In addition to being easier, I wonder if large spaces, deforested and mowed down for roads and cars and bikes, for easier (read: less) on-foot movement, are sending us a message. It seems clear that many human movements are reflexive, and that walking is reflexive, but perhaps those reflexes only express themselves fully when the human is in a more natural habitat, where nature—wilderness, temperature, hunger, fear of isolation—facilitates the body's forward movement in an organic way. Maybe a kid out of nature will behave differently from a kid in nature, simply because nature—dirt, grass, weeds, lumps, bumps, wind—is facilitating behaviors in ways a parent couldn't possibly recreate outside of nature, despite endless trying.

I don't know much about human psychology, but I do know that when given a wide-open, asphalted space, my son was less apt to move forward steadily. And when presented with a more narrow, complex trail, he not only moved forward steadily, he did so screaming with joy. Or maybe that was me.

TREE BONES

You can learn a lot about the human body by studying trees. This is what I love most about biomechanics—that it applies to all living things, not only to humans.

My brother-in-law is a badass in many ways, none so much as in his knowledge of plants, but I thought I'd tell him something he didn't know about trees. I said, "Hey, bro, you see how that tree's branches go from big to small to smaller to smallest? That branching geometry is very specific—it's called *fractal*."

I was showing off.

I rambled on about Leonardo da Vinci and how trees rarely splinter under their weight, even in high winds, because they *sense* the wind as they grow and adjust their shape to the loads to stay strong in that particular environment.[4] This also explains why trees belonging to a particular species look similar enough to be recognizable as that species, but why they, like humans, don't all have the same exact shape, and why (or is it how?) the branches of a particular tree aren't shaped exactly like those of its tree-brothers or tree-sisters. Or tree-parents. Or tree-aunts and tree-uncles.

Just like a drafting cyclist will experience a bout of cycling differently from a lead cyclist, who's bearing the brunt of the air, trees just inches apart will each experience the environment differently, moment to moment, and therefore branch differently. The variance in their shapes doesn't imply that they work differently from other trees, but the opposite: that trees adapt in a very predictable way to their experience. A tree's final shape is determined by the loads that it experiences as it's growing.

And seriously, if they taught stuff like this in school, wouldn't we all have been more interested in geometry and biology?

Then my brother-in-law OH BROed me. An OH BRO is where you say something cool and the OH BROer immediately tells you about something they did or know that is cooler than what you just said. I have a horrible habit of OH BROing, which is why it kills me to be OH BROed. And just so you know, you are now going to recognize OH BROs and OH BROers everywhere. You're welcome.

My OH BROing bro said that this is why many trees grown in nurseries have branches that are too long and thin, unable to survive once introduced into nature. And also there was research showing that simulating "natural movement" (i.e., loading the trees multiple times a day while they're growing) resulted in trees with shorter and thicker branches compared to a control group.[5]

Well, bro, if you're going to OH BRO me with MINDBLOW-INGLY AWESOME information, then feel free to do so anytime.

It all made so much sense, and I love it when tree and human science reconcile. Humans have mechanoreceptors and their shape adapts to how they move; why wouldn't trees behave similarly?

Early bone has a reflexive tendency to grow. Meaning your bones, like trees, will grow because they contain an internal program to do so. But the shape a bone takes is not only reflexive, it is also dependent on what your body is doing *while* it is growing longer (or bigger or thicker or whatever).

When physical anthropologists compare bones of hunter-gatherer populations to the skeletons of more modern, agriculture-based peoples, it appears that the shape of our bones, like trees, is affected by the quantities and qualities of movement we have done to date.

Beyond traumatic and often sports-related risks and injuries, we aren't taught to think of our bones as being influenced by things like how we behave, and when it comes to investigating the very prolific (and expensive) issues associated with bone health, it's rarely mentioned that how you loaded them while growing might be an important place to begin an investigation.

When you're looking at the tall, thin branches of an indoor tree, it's easy to see that this tree wouldn't fare well in an outdoor mechanical environment of wind and snow and interactions with animals. Similarly, when we look at the osteoporotic bones of 200 million women throughout the world,[6] the shape of them indicates a future inability to withstand the mechanical environment created by movement. The bones of these women's hips aren't strong enough to bear the weight of their bodies and so they crack, like a tree in the wind.

We've identified the problem as the state of the bone, deciding that it's too porous and too inflexible and thus prone to shattering. But what if instead we focused on the state of the bone as the result of a lifetime of loading behavior in a particular habitat?

When I walk through the woods, I not only use my body more (and enjoy the resultant bone stimulation) but by paying attention to trees, I also experience how much I am a part of nature. Perhaps experiencing and studying the natural world should go hand in hand. Perhaps closing ourselves off in our houses and cars and malls and schools has shaped not only our bodies but also our perception that we fall outside of the natural laws governing everything—especially those natural processes modeling and remodeling physical structures. Staying indoors may impact the way we think, but not how we function: we are shaped by the forces we experience. We've removed the wind and, likewise, the strength to withstand it.

---

4. Krieger, Kim. 2011. "Leonardo's Formula Explains Why Trees Don't Splinter." *Science*, November 14. <sciencemag.org/news/2011/11/leonardos-formula-explains-why-trees-dont-splinter>

5. Stokes, Alexia. 1994. "Responses of Young Trees to Wind: Effects on Root Architecture and Anchorage Strength." (Doctoral thesis.) York, England: University of York. <etheses.whiterose.ac.uk/2438/1/DX184141.pdf>

6. Kanis, J.A. (on behalf of the World Health Organization Scientific Group). 2007. WHO Technical Report. University of Sheffield, UK: 66.

Additional Sources

Chaney, William R. 2001. "How Wind Affects Trees." *Indiana Woodland Steward* 10(1). <woodlandsteward.squarespace.com/storage/past-issues/windaffe.htm>

Moulia, Bruno, Catherine Coutand, and Jean-Louis Julien. (2015) 2016. "Mechanosensitive Control of Plant Growth: Bearing the Load, Sensing, Transducing, and Responding." *Frontiers in Plant Science* 6(52). PMC. Web. May 22.

A MATTER OF PERSPECTIVE

Trees are shaped by the wind, but here's the thing: the wind is also shaped by the trees. A wind heading into a forest will hit all the trees differently, but the trees are also hitting the wind. The wind is not constant, and everything affects everything else.

I can say that a river is moving in a particular direction, but if you get up close to it and look, you'll see that while all of it eventually moves that way, the water also swirls around, heading faster or slower than, and perpendicular or even opposite to the direction the river as a whole is flowing. Same with the wind. I can tell you how fast it's going and in what direction, but if you measure that same wind amongst the trees, it's moving all over the place, in different directions and at different speeds than what you measured very scientifically in a single place.

To measure all the ways in which a particular volume of water or air can move in its journey isn't always feasible, but to *know* and note that you've assumed an easy measure to simplify the behavior of a river or a wind—or a body or a cell—is necessary. Clarifying, if only to yourself, that your understanding of something is limited to an unmoving, non-interacting version of that something helps keep perspective—especially when your job is trying to figure out and describe how things work and behave in real life; that is, out of a vacuum and in their lifelong environment.

WET BONES

Human bones are so similar to trees, I've always thought of young bones as being flexible or "wet" like green twigs, and old bones as being brittle and dry, like dead branches.

I suppose my thinking was influenced by some courses I took on injury. Often the breaking of a very supple (usually young) bone is called a "greenstick" or "greentwig" fracture because flexible bone fractures sort of like a green twig does when you try to snap it (if you've never tried to snap a green twig, know that despite lots of trying to break it, it only slightly splinters or fractures on one side while the rest of the twig stays intact). An older, almost-dead branch of the same size would snap under the same forces. In my mind, bones were either wet and supple or dry and brittle.

But I also "knew" that unlike trees, the break-resistance of bone isn't really due to its wetness or dryness. Bone strength is a matter of density, and it's greater density of mineral that helps bone resist breaks. But here's what's always bothered me: current bone science states that healthy bone is flexible, but also that it has more mineral density, *which would make it harder.* So how can both be true? For a long time I was confused as to how one aspect of a healthy bone (more mineral mass) could be exclusive of another aspect of a healthy bone (flexibility). Biomechanics should line up across all living things, and in this case it didn't.

When data seems to be in conflict with other data, it's usually due to a problem with a basic model/assumption. In this case, the issue I was having stemmed from the general assumption that minerals were solids (the definition is now apparently under debate, but at one point "naturally occurring inorganic solid" was the definition of a mineral).

Enter new findings: Bone minerals come with goo. In between what we've been calling bone minerals is "shock-absorbing goo"[7]—goo that allows these minerals to slide over each other without sticking (the cited article uses a great analogy of how two pieces of glass with water between them would slide over each other). When your bone is less porous, it holds more goo, making your bone move with less resistance (i.e., it's more flexible) and when your bone is more porous, this goo leaks out. So you're left with just the hard minerals that can't slide over each other. From the article cited above:

> "Bone mineral was thought to be closely related to this substance called hydroxyapatite. But what we've shown is that a large part of bone mineral—possibly as much as half of it, in fact—is made up of this goo, where citrate is binding like a gel between mineral crystals," said Dr. Melinda Duer, who led the study.

Bones with more mineral density are more "wet." Mineral density and flexibility and resistance to fracture go hand in hand. Human bone behaves similarly to trees, and all is right with the world. Or at least with my understanding of biomechanics, today.

---

7. University of Cambridge. 2014. "Shock-Absorbing 'Goo' Discovered in Bone." ScienceDaily. <sciencedaily.com/releases/2014/03/140324154013.htm>

Additional Sources

Davies, Erika, Karin H. Muller, Wai Ching Wong, Chris J. Pickard, David G. Reid, Jeremy N. Skepper, and Melinda J. Duer. 2014. "Citrate Bridges between Mineral Platelets in Bone." *Proceedings of the National Academy of Sciences*. doi:10.1073/pnas.1315080111.

MYOPIC

The "sitting is the new smoking" campaign really highlights how much time we spend sitting in chairs. Sitting isn't good for us, the research clearly shows, and thus health enthusiasts have begun their migration out of their chairs and into the standing position. But what's really the problem with sitting in a chair? Is it the repetitive positioning of the body and the adaptations to that position? Is it that the chair limits the use of the knees, hips, and ankles, in that if you were to take a seat on the ground, you would have articulated all of your joints to a much fuller extent and used your muscles to control the weight of your body over a much greater distance? Is it that when you're sitting, you're not moving—and your physiology has to deal with the consequences of maintaining a dynamic system in which many parts have ground to a halt? It's likely that "the problem with sitting" is all of these, yet the takeaway "solution" has seemed to be simply "stand more." (This, in my opinion, is the predictable outcome of a sedentary culture looking at the problem of sitting—identifying the problem as the *wrong type* of stillness, and not as stillness itself.)

There's no escaping the reality of it: our bodies are shaped both by what we do and what we don't do. Time spent sitting is also time spent not doing all other things. Likewise, time spent looking at things less than two feet from our faces—computers, phone screens, iPads, and books—is time spent not looking to all distances beyond two feet.

When you look at things close to your face, your eye changes the shape of its parts to be able to focus on them. From page 151 of my favorite anatomy book, *Clinical Anatomy Made Ridiculously Simple*, by Stephen Goldberg:

Contraction of muscles in the ciliary ring narrows the diameter of the ring. This decreases the tension of the zonules, and releases the tension on the lens. The lens then thickens leading to a stronger focus (accommodation). Thus, accommodation is the process in which the ciliary muscles contract, thereby relaxing tension on the lens and enabling one to focus closer on the object.

Got it? No? BUT IT'S RIDICULOUSLY SIMPLE! It's not, actually, but here's how accommodation—the necessary tensing of your ciliary muscles in order to see close up—happens.

The ciliary muscle is a ring of smooth muscle that surrounds the lens of the eye. Similar to the walls of a blood vessel that can contract to become a smaller tube and relax to become a larger one, when ciliary muscle contracts, it measures a smaller diameter than when it's relaxed.

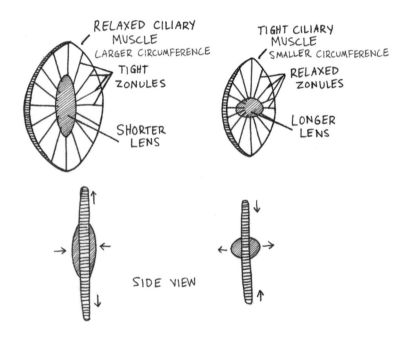

RELAXED CILIARY MUSCLE
LARGER CIRCUMFERENCE
TIGHT ZONULES
SHORTER LENS

TIGHT CILIARY MUSCLE
SMALLER CIRCUMFERENCE
RELAXED ZONULES
LONGER LENS

SIDE VIEW

"Zonules" are fibers that surround the lens like guy-wires, connecting it to the ciliary muscle. Because the lens of the eye is connected to the ciliary muscles via the zonules, the shape of the lens depends on the circumference of the ciliary ring. When the muscle relaxes—(see left-hand images on page 66)—the motion places the zonules under tension, and the zonules in turn pull on the edges of the lens, thinning it. When the ciliary muscle contracts, it releases the tension in the lens, which allows the lens to thicken and become longer.

To read this book, your ciliary muscles contracted, allowing the lens to increase its center thickness. If you looked up from your book and to the closest wall, your eyes would disaccommodate—relaxing the ciliary muscles, tightening the zonules, and causing the lens to reduce its central thickness, effectively focusing light onto the retina from a further distance. If you were to look at a wall beyond the wall where we last left your gaze, your eyes would disaccommodate even more. Meaning, to keep things from being too ridiculously simple, there aren't only two sizes (read: positions) of the ciliary body or lens. Every distance between "close up" and "far away" correlates to a certain amount of tension in the ciliary muscle. Because the muscle contraction and relaxation controls the focusing of the lens, your eye is able to focus from far distance to close reading distance smoothly.

To utilize the full range of motion of your biceps muscles, you would have to curl your arm all the way up and all the way down. Similarly, using the full range of motion of your eye requires that you look over *all the distances*.

Alongside the development of our technology-based culture has been a tremendous increase in the development of myopia in children. It's not that surprising. With technology comes a lot of *near-work* (the research term for time spent writing, reading, looking at tablets, phones, and computer screens), and thus research focused first on the obvious candidate for myopia—too much looking up close.[8] But, just as sitting isn't only a position, *near-work* isn't only a position. "Near-work," it seems, is also "lots of time spent inside."

> Discovering that spending more time outdoors reduces the risk of the onset of myopia represents a major advance in our understanding of refractive error. But, we need to figure out what's so good about more time outdoors—exercise, brighter light, vitamin D synthesis, or some combination.[9]

Of course, exercise and light and vitamin D are all aspects of being outside, but so is distance-looking. Looking at things far away is the only way to release a tense ciliary ring within an eyeball, thus taking the elongating pressure off the eye. But despite it being a simple explanation for at least one contributing factor to the myopia issue, "distance-looking" isn't on the list. (I'm thinking that because they've eliminated one distance, near-work, as a cause, scientists don't think another distance would be worth investigation.)

Delineation is the process of defining variables as precisely as possible. It would be more clear to define "near-work" with numbers—say, 0–2 feet (0–0.6 meters). Better yet, distances can be converted into a percentage of the total distance over which the human eye could focus. There's debate around how far the eye can see, but most recent estimates figure it (mathematically) to be about

1.6 miles (2.6 kilometers).[10] (An interesting note and one I feel supports my larger point in this section: There are many studies on close ranges of the eye and accommodation, and very few on how much the ciliary body can relax, "what happens" when you look at distances atypical of chronic indoor living, and how far the eye can see—the difficulty of finding a mile uninterrupted by structures being cited as a limiting factor to testing.)

If we want to keep in mind the eye's capacity for distance vision, then we could convert "near-work" to a percentage of that capacity. If we (under)estimate the distance one could see, unobstructed, toward the horizon to be one mile (1.6 kilometers) and convert the mile measure into the smaller units used to measure near-work (5,280 feet/1,609 meters), then research findings could accurately read, "Myopia is rapidly developing in populations that have recently started limiting their eyes' use to less than a half of 1 percent of their eyes' range of focus, by frequently focusing for near work—0.04 percent of the range—and the rest of the time looking to a distance allowed indoors (the wall behind your iPad is still only 20 feet away!)—0.4 percent of that range." The numbers show how serious the issue is. And whether or not our lack of using all of the movements natural for the eye is at play when it comes to solving myopia, these numbers give our eyeball-sedentarism a level of gravitas that shouldn't go unexplored by researchers.

Like the branches of a tree adjusting their shape to the wind, myopia seems to be the very unmysterious adaptation of an eyeball being shaped, extremely, by the forces placed upon it while growing (which can also include forces brought about by high blood sugar, but I'll save that for another time).

But here's why I don't think eye researchers are considering distance-looking: A life spent almost entirely inside is typical for our culture, and likely common for those humans developing the research questions. "Indoors" is not an abnormal state for the eye if you've spent your entire life there, but tech devices are new. And so, we began with the abnormal-to-us state of the eye—looking at a lot of tech devices—rather than the abnormal-in-human-history state of the eye—looking at things indoors all the time. Had accommodation been delineated mathematically, it would be more clear to everyone how similar the eye's use for near-work is to the eye's use while focusing the typical distances found indoors. If never looking beyond the walls of your house doesn't seem unnatural to you, then it might not occur to you that being outdoors—the normal habitat for the eyeball and one that the eye has evolved to for millennia—allows for an entirely different use. It could also be that there are no easy-to-access structure-free mile-long distances over which to measure how far an eye can see. Either way, this potential limitation of myopia research seems to be brought about by a culture that has set itself up to not see that far ahead.

P.S. Clearly, the vision-related puns in this essay were coincidental.

P.P.S. I said on page 67 that looking long distances was the only way to release the ciliary body, but there's a drug—atropine[11]—which paralyzes the ciliary body for up to two weeks at a time, inhibiting accommodation. This is what's currently being used to prevent myopia in some cases. So, there's that, or simply going outside and looking at things that are far away.

8. Huang, Hsiu-Mei, Dolly Shuo-Teh Chang, Pei-Chang Wu. 2015. "The Association between Near Work Activities and Myopia in Children—A Systematic Review and Meta-Analysis." *PLOS ONE*. October 15. <dx.doi.org/10.1371/journal.pone.0140419>

9. Mutti, Donald O., OD, PhD. 2013. "Time Outdoors and Myopia: A Case for Vitamin D?" *Optometry Times*. <optometrytimes.modernmedicine.com/optom-etrytimes/content/tags/cleere-study/time-outdoors-and-myopia-case-vita-min-d>

10. Krisciunas, Kevin, and Don Carona. 2015. "At What Distance Can the Human Eye Detect a Candle Flame?" Research paper. Cornell University Library. <arXiv:1507.06270>

11. American Academy of Ophthalmology. 2015. "Nearsighteness Progression in Children Slowed Down by Medicated Eye Drops." MedicalXpress, November 17. <medicalxpress.com/news/2015-11-nearsightedness-children-medicat-ed-eye.html>

YOU SPEAK HOW YOU ARE

In 2008 the *Oxford Junior Dictionary* (a dictionary geared to seven-year-olds) updated their text, removing many nature words.

They were: acorn, adder, allotment, almond, apricot, ash, ass (come on. What are seven-year-olds going to look up and snicker at now?), bacon (um, what?), beaver, beech, beetroot, blackberry, blacksmith, bloom (Orlando), bluebell, bramble, bran, bray, bridle, brook, budgerigar (had to look it up, in my 2007 *Oxford Junior Dictionary*), bullock (Sandra), buttercup, canary, canter, carnation, catkin (again, had to look it up), cauliflower, cheetah, chestnut, clover, colt, conker (what you do to your sister when she knocks down your blocks on purpose), corgi (with apologies to my grandma and the Queen, whom I've recently learned are not the same person), county, cowslip, crocus, cygnet, dandelion, diesel, doe, drake, fern, ferret, fungus, gerbil, goldfish (dead), gooseberry, gorse (offspring of a goat and a horse), guinea pig, hamster, hazel, hazelnut, heather, heron, herring, holly, horse chestnut, ivy, kingfisher, lavender, lark, leek, leopard, liquorice, lobster, magpie, manger, marzipan (remind me to tell you about my eighth birthday party, when the Queen—I mean, my grandma—made me a gorgeous princess marzipan cake and it tasted horrible to my seven-year-old palate—good riddance, marzipan!), melon, minnow, mint, mistletoe, mussel, nectar, nectarine, newt (this one is breaking my heart), oats, otter, ox, oyster, pansy, panther (pink), parsnip, pasture, pelican, piglet, plaice, poodle (I'm fine with the removal of this one), poppy, porcupine, porpoise, porridge, poultry, primrose, prune, radish, raven, rhubarb, sheaf, spaniel, spinach, starling, stoat, stork, sycamore, terrapin (the best way to open a birthday present), thrush, tulip, turnip, vine, violet, walnut, weasel, willow, wren.

According to an official statement from Oxford University Press on the matter, "[Our dictionaries] reflect the language that children are encouraged to use in the classroom as required by the national curriculum. This ensures they remain relevant and beneficial for children's education."

Some words that were added: analogue, blog, broadband, MP3 player (are the kids listening to MP3s again, on players?), voicemail, attachment, database, export, chatroom, bullet point, cut and paste (does sticking the words together really change the meaning that dramatically?), celebrity, tolerant, vandalism, negotiate, interdependent, creep, citizenship, childhood, conflict, common sense, debate, EU, drought, brainy, boisterous, cautionary tale, bilingual, bungee jumping, committee, compulsory, cope, democratic, allergic, biodegradable, emotion, dyslexic, donate, endangered, Euro.

Oxford University Press got some flack for removing the nature words, receiving many petitions and letters requesting these words be let back in, but as it noted, Oxford University Press does not shape language—it reflects it. If children aren't using nature words any longer because their lives no longer include nature, it isn't the fault of a dictionary company.

In a seemingly unrelated event, the *Journal of Obesity Research and Clinical Practice* published a study[12] that explains that in studies where people report their calorie and daily exercise and activities, it appears people are more obese than their calorie consumption warrants. We keep assuming these people are underreporting their food intake because we "know" that weight is determined by a "calorie-in, calorie-out" equation, but maybe it's not that simple. Recent studies show that hormonal changes brought about by physiology-altering habits (intrinsic) or environmental toxins (extrinsic) may be altering the disposition of calories in the body.

Or if studies came in diagram form:

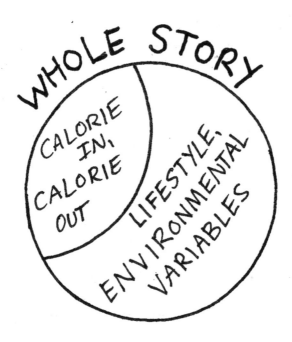

The paper goes on to talk about researched variables associated with higher BMI, the variables including:

- Persistent organic pollutants
- Pharmaceutical prescriptions associated with weight gain
- Lack of varying ambient temperature
- Inadequate amount of sleep
- Low calcium
- Bacteriome/microbiota

Says the paper, "As well, the majority of agricultural beef cattle are given exogenous sex steroids in order to increase weight gain and feeding efficiency. Although there are concerns that this may influence human health, more research in this area is needed."

These seemingly unrelated events connected themselves in my mind when I read a headline placed on an article about this study: "Millennials, Gen Y Need to Eat Less, Work Out More to Stave Off Obesity, Researchers Say."[13] Or, if headlines came in diagram form:

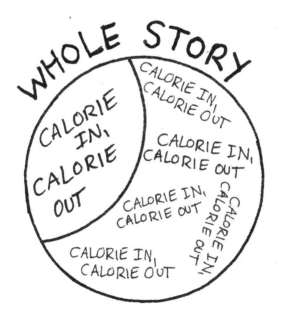

Um, what?

The research article doesn't state anything about people needing to approach their body mass index (in itself a significantly flawed measure) through a caloric perspective. What it is stating is that it might be more than calories eaten or burned affecting the current shape of your body. From the article:

> Kuk further explains that our body weight is impacted by our lifestyle and environment, such as medication use, environmental pollutants, genetics, timing of food intake, stress, gut bacteria and even nighttime light exposure. "Ultimately, maintaining a healthy body weight is now more challenging than ever."

Although it might feel like the problem, obesity is in fact a symptom. The problem is still being identified. Body fat issues have been reduced to putting-too-much-in-your-mouth problems, and certainly, what one puts in one's mouth is playing a role, as is the amount/rate/way one expends energy. But these aren't the only variables at play. To continue with this narrow view is to assume that our physiologically taxing habitats are unchangeable, with the only solution being to eat fewer calories and to exercise. *Not* to eat higher-quality foods with a more suitable overall macronutrient and micronutrient profile, *not* to get more rest and remove the chemicals from your home, office, and schools, *not* to stop overdosing on antibiotics and antibacterial products, and *not* to get out of your home on a daily basis and get into the dirt. But instead, continue to live the same lifestyle that resulted in the problem while following the insufficient prescription *harder*. I used to suggest skipping the headline and reading the full article instead, but these days, I bypass the articles entirely and go straight to the research being reported on.

So these articles, on the loss of nature words and the obesity research, swirled together in my head because they shared a common thread: symptoms.

Many framed the first problem as being Oxford University Press removing certain words from the dictionary, and not these words becoming obsolete in our current society (the assumption being that society is a single composite of people who go to school, learn a particular curriculum, get particular jobs, follow specific rules, and desire the same outcomes). The language in the *Oxford Junior Dictionary* is a symptom of the language we actually use, which is a symptom of how we have chosen to live.

Similarly, we think of obesity and many of our other health issues as the problem, but what if we framed them as a symptom instead? I continue to see over and over again in research of the affluent ailments—cardiovascular disease, cancer, osteoporosis, myopia, obesity—that the variables listed as potential risk factors are scenarios brought about by our attempt to live *outside of nature,* inside walls that limit how far we can see, chairs that prevent our hips and knees from bending all the way to get us to the floor, and thermostats that keep our body temperature at a constant with no physiological work involved. We can either treat symptoms— in this case by protesting the loss of words and an institution's failure to preserve seemingly obsolete vocabulary, or by continuing to sit unmoving in our houses, eating few calories and boosting the intensity of our one hour of exercise—or we can address the problem, and live in a way that keeps natural language, and natural movement, relevant to us. Either way, dictionaries and article head-lines don't give us permission to speak of or move through nature; those choices are ours alone.

---

12. Brown, Ruth E., Arya M. Sharma, Chris I. Ardern, Pedi Mirdamadi, Paul Mirdamadi, and Jennifer L. Kuk. 2015. "Secular Differences in the Association Between Caloric Intake, Macronutrient Intake, and Physical Activity with Obesity." *Obesity Research and Clinical Practice.* <obesityresearchclinicalpractice. com/article/S1871-403X%2815%2900121-0/abstract>

13. York University. "Millennials, Gen Y Need to Eat Less, Work Out More to Stave Off Obesity, Researchers Say: The Study Results Suggest that if You Are 25, You'd Have to Eat Even Less and Exercise More than Those Older." *ScienceDaily*. <sciencedaily.com/releases/2015/09/150921133654.htm>

Additional Sources

Baillie-Hamilton, P. F. 2002. "Chemical Toxins: a Hypothesis to Explain the Global Obesity Epidemic." *Journal of Alternative and Complementary Medicine* 8: 185–192.

Chaput, J.-P., J.-P. Després, C. Bouchard, and A. Tremblay. 2008. "The Association Between Sleep Duration and Weight Gain in Adults: A 6-Year Prospective Study from the Quebec Family Study." *Sleep* 31: 517–523.

Gangwisch, J., D. Malaspina, B. Boden-Albala, and S. Heymsfield. 2005. "Inadequate Sleep as a Risk Factor for Obesity: Analyses of the NHANES I." *Sleep* 28: 1289–1296.

Keith, S. W., D. T. Redden, P. T. Katzmarzyk et al. 2006. "Putative Contributors to the Secular Increase in Obesity: Exploring the Roads Less Traveled." *International Journal of Obesity* 30: 1585–1594.

Knutson, K. 2012. "Does Inadequate Sleep Play a Role in Vulnerability to Obesity?" *American Journal of Human Biology* 24: 361–371.

Lind, P. M., D.-H. Lee, D. R. Jacobs et al. 2013. "Circulating Levels of Persistent Organic Pollutants Are Related to Retrospective Assessment of Life-Time Weight Change." *Chemosphere* 90: 998–1004.

Lusk, J., J. Roosen, and J. Fox. 2003. "Demand for Beef from Cattle Administered Growth Hormones or Fed Genetically Modified Corn: A Comparison of Consumers in France, Germany, the United Kingdom, and the United States." *American Journal of Agricultural Economics* 85: 16–29.

Nieuwdorp, M., P. W. Gilijamse, N. Pai, and L. M. Kaplan. 2014. "Role of the Microbiome in Energy Regulation and Metabolism." *Gastroenterology* 146(6): 1525-1533.

OUTDOOR SCHOOL

Like many families, we had to decide what to do about educating our kids. Like many parents, we began thinking, "What will we do??" when our first kid was three hours old. Flash forward one more kid and five years later: our kids have been enrolled in a nature preschool for two years now.

Choosing nature school for my kids was one part reduction and one part intuition. My "research!" brain went to the data. I read studies that showed that outdoor time was protective against nearsightedness; that sitting the bulk of the day, how should I say, isn't good for the body; that dirt and fresh air and vitamin D *are* good for the body; that the experience of a variety of temperatures is beneficial to the body; that the interaction with phytoncides (airborne chemicals emitted from plants that protect them from rotting and insects, and that seem to boost white blood cells and reduce stress) was beneficial to the body.

Then there were the implicit parts of nature school that I found to be of benefit: that having no chairs could mean less restrictive, all-day movement; that plant knowledge—the recognition of edible, medicinal, and native plants—was a "natural language" acquired most easily at an early age; that the lack of a building meant no nature had to be destroyed to house our children's education; that no fuel had to be consumed to keep our kids comfortable for the duration of a school day, etc.

But it was the other stuff—the intuitive stuff—that really drove our decision. My husband and I felt, deeply, that there was a value in learning to be comfortable without comforts, to be comfortable in nature. We wanted our kids to have a relationship with nature, and we felt that they could exist in nature—they could *be* nature—by better understanding it. We felt that through understanding nature, they would better understand themselves.

Two years into their schooling, our children's understanding of nature has far exceeded our expectations and, frankly, our own personal knowledge about the natural world. While I have a long list of facts about nature that includes the names of plants and the mechanics by which they reproduce, our children have developed a functional relationship with nature itself, which includes the development of the physiology necessary for regular long-term exposure in nature (see the photo of my daughter's ankle range of motion on page 53 for just one example of this).

One does not adapt to facts about fresh air and the names of plants and the stages of plant reproduction and the language of birds in the same way they can adapt to being in the fresh air; touching, climbing through, and sometimes eating many plants; and experiencing bird calls in the environment that prompts them. Parts of their bodies have shifted to better facilitate a relationship between them and the land they engage with for hours each week, and thus they have more than just knowledge of nature; they're wise to it.

I don't know if evidence trumps intuition, or if evidence is even meant to be used when approaching social issues like how best to educate children, but in the end, both evidence and intuition pointed us, yet again, toward nature, and nature school and the foundation it would set for more movement and flexibility in our children's bodies and minds. Like many parents, we're working hard to keep up with our kids!

For more information on outdoor school, nature in education, and getting more nature into your and your family's lives when nature school isn't an option, see Appendix 1.

DEAR KATY

Q WHAT DO YOU LOVE MOST ABOUT BIOMECHANICS?

A For me, the biggest draw to biomechanics was its efficiency as a course of study. Like most going to college, I had the opportunity to study a single subject, but by picking biomechanics, it opened up an understanding of many other fields as it provided a foundation in the basic inner workings of all natural things, not only the body. Biomechanics, as it is currently taught in universities, should really be written bioMECHANICS because principles of biology make almost zero appearance in biomechanical models, especially at introductory levels. After many years of research and reading beyond my program's curriculum, I now think of myself as a BIOmechanist in that I consider principles of evolutionary biology, general biology, and ecology to come up with the most robust biomechanical model I can. This is what I love about biomechanics. Like the body, it's hugely adaptable to many courses of thought.

Q AREN'T YOU WORRIED THAT NATURE SCHOOL WON'T OFFER A FOUNDATION IN THE TECHNOLOGICAL SKILLS OUR CHILDREN WILL LIKELY NEED IN THE FUTURE?

A My dad is almost ninety years old and grew up working on farms and spending lots of time outside. He was one of the first people to fly a plane, fix televisions, and learn to control air traffic—all requiring a proficiency in technology that hadn't been around while he was growing up. His current apartment has three computers (yes, he uses them all) and he is known to send selfies from his iPhone. Similarly, I grew up on a farm with no computers and do the bulk of my work, successfully, on the computer.

There is no data at this time that implies an early specialization in technology is necessary for proficient, prolific use later in life. The jobs of the future will include technology, but the fluency in nature offers foundational skills that will be necessary for growing food, restoring wilderness, protecting the remaining wilderness, and moving through wilderness with competence. As these skills are lost, their value increases tremendously. I believe my children's time in outdoor school will not only prime them physically to endure a technology-profuse life should they choose it, but also, perhaps, give them an understanding of the question that will likely consume the future: how can we continue to sustain a human population on the planet (i.e., how can the entire human population continue to eat and breathe given the environmental impact of many people and many technologies)?

Q   I WAS TAUGHT TO STAY ON THE PATH IN WILDERNESS AREAS OUT OF RESPECT FOR THE MICRO-ENVIRONMENTS. WOULDN'T EVERYONE GOING OFF ESTABLISHED TRAILS WRECK WILD AREAS?

A   There are many people working hard to reestablish wildlife— plants and animals—in areas that have been destroyed for whatever reason. Of course, we should respect this work by keeping off new life to give it a chance to succeed. In this respect, I'm entirely in support of restoration work and think "Keep Off This

Area" signs should be heeded. However, because we see ourselves as things that exist out of nature, we're setting up nature as something that functions as a museum or as a vacation from the other, non-nature place we live, rather than stressing the essentialness of it to our ability to thrive.

Whether or not we stray off a trail or pick up a stick while in the woods, we leave more than a trace on wilderness all day long. Our traces are all the terribly made clothes in our closet that we buy weekly because we like new clothes (and I'm not even going into the sociological impact of supporting sweatshops here because other humans seem to fall outside of nature, so…), and the plastic water bottles and paper cups we buy and toss multiple times a day. They're the bulk discount meat we buy cheap, or the hamburgers we drive through to order. I made healthy smoothies from coconut milk for years without being aware that it contained seaweed. In fact, a lot of things most people use daily, like cosmetics and shampoo and industrialized beef, utilize seaweed—a vital habitat and nourishment to marine life. Our traces are the fuel necessary to get lanolin, pulled from sheep's wool, to process it into vitamin D for our fortified milk or orange juice—because we spend so much time inside. They're the plastic toys for sale in the national parks, made possible by destroying nature elsewhere, to remind you of that time you went into nature and it was gorgeous, wasn't it?

I used to be entirely unaware of how we stomp all over nature all day long—until I actually engaged as a part of nature. I've found that by prioritizing interactions with nature and wilderness, I consume less, eat more mindfully, sleep more, use less fossil fuel, recycle, and generally make better, more considerate choices. I love our national park areas, but I can see that the framing of nature areas as national, and something we must protect for a nation, is a mindset that easily leads to a nationalistic "environmentalism"—one that doesn't address how okay we are with nature being destroyed elsewhere. For this reason, I'd like to see nature programs engage humans in nature, work to restore a functional and sustainable relationship between humans and the rest of the world, and use language that defines nature as a global phenomenon and not a national one.

I can definitely see how a lot of people going off-path in a nature preserve would result in the destruction of a small area. It's definitely a capacity issue, but is it too many people or is it that we have such a small area allotted for human/nature interactions? Maybe it's that the bulk of us, even the conservation-minded, prefer to be sedentary and inside. The nature destroyed daily for our comfortable, sedentary lifestyle is staggering. At every turn, our comfort and lack of movement are the issues that, if we each choose to address them *alongside* better stewardship, can bring about radical improvement for nature and all its animals, including humans.

Additional Sources

Leschin-Hoar, Clare. 2014. "Help for Kelp—Seaweed Slashers See Harvesting Cuts Coming." *Scientific American*, May 14. <scientificamerican.com/article/help-for-kelp-seaweed-slashers-see-harvesting-cuts-coming>

FOOD *moves*

The major problems in the world are the result of the difference between how nature works and the way people think.

–GREGORY BATESON

Hunger is nature's personal trainer and a relentless one at that. When animals live in nature, hunger gets them up and moving throughout the day, looking for food. For millions of years, hunger was efficient in that a single signal served animal bodies in two ways: it got them food and it got them movement.

For we human animals who have altered our environment so that food and water appear with ease, the move/eat signal is easily squelched. This leaves us with bodies rich in nutritional input and malnourished in mechanical loads—a situation where disease springs forth with ease.

Because we've grown up in a time and place where almost all movement has been entirely outsourced, we don't recognize the essentialness of it. Our lack of movement is easily catered to by a cumulative mass of technologies that have become normal. Said another way, we've mistaken no longer needing food-related movements to get food for no longer needing the movements themselves.

We have grown up totally unaware of the movements being done on our behalf to facilitate life in our unmoving bodies. This section deals with perhaps the most fundamental movements we've outsourced—those necessary to make nature edible for our survival.

MUST WORK FOR FOOD

Food does not grow in nature. Plants and animals occur in nature, and you can turn these items into food with mechanical work, but without that work, there is no food. If you've been eating without doing much work, my question for you is: Who and where is your food coming from?

In the natural world, food and movement are organically related; how you eat is based on your ability to get and prepare your food. By being directly involved at every step throughout your life, you maintain the skills and physique necessary to continue to cultivate, obtain, and process your own food.

Historically, the work (i.e., the forces created by human movement) necessary to eat included not only the hunting and gathering of food, but also the mashing, banging, rubbing, beating, tearing, pounding, soaking, spreading, turning, and hanging it took to make things growing in nature *edible*. Most of the food we now use to make our meals—even "whole ingredients" like nut and coconut flours, the oils, milks, and syrups we pour with ease, the meats cut with precision, and the veggies cleaned and separated for our convenience—has been processed. Not in the chemistry-lab, "I created this edible item by putting different chemicals together," kind of way, but a, "Hey, a whole bunch of people somewhere else just performed fourteen hours of labor for very little money so I could have these 'whole foods' to cook for my meal, thanks for that" kind of way.

Natural movement has gone sexy. Running, tackling, sprinting, climbing, crawling, leaping, and choreographed feats of athleticism are on the rise. I get it: everyone wants to behave the way they imagine a traditional hunter did/does. Our society likes to extract "the best" of something ("the best" being based on our cultural conditioning, and usually equaling "the awesomest") and then consume a ton of it. We eat the muscle of an animal while disregarding what we perceive as the lesser parts: the heads, hooves, skin, and organs. Similarly, we've cast aside the non-grand motions required for us to eat. The digging of tubers, pummeling of acorns, shelling of nuts, plucking of berries from their bushes, climbing of and balancing in trees to gather nuts and fruits, the miles and miles and miles of slow-paced walking in a group of mixed ages, filled with frequent bends and squats to gather food which is then carried farther, for miles and miles.

It's ironic that we've become so unaware or dismissive of gathering and processing movements, when it's these subtler food-related movements that made it feasible for bodies to perform the awesome hunting movements we admire. The environment of traditional, awesome physical feats *always* included the movements we now underestimate. The difference is that in today's world, we seek the grand performances while demanding someone else, out of sight, do the mundane tasks on our behalf. By seeking only a portion of all the movements available to us, we're undernourished in movement. Put another way, we're full up on movement steak but missing all the movement leaves, fruits, seeds, and roots.

THOSE OTHER NUTRIENTS

Eating is a phenomenon we all engage in to survive. We've always eaten for energy, even before science told us that's what we were doing, but it wasn't until fairly recently, during the last five hundred years or so, that science said we were also eating for nutrients— those unique chemical compounds found in food, without which we wouldn't be able to fully function. Our understanding of how food works is really in its infancy; we are still in the process of isolating and describing all the parts included in the phenomenon we call food.

Perhaps the most significant contribution I can make to the discussion about food-related parts is this: When you chew your food—when you move the food with your tongue and teeth and jaw and skull bones and muscles—your tongue and teeth and jaw and skull bones and muscles are being moved right back. When you eat, you get more out of the food than what's contained within it; there's value to be gained in terms of the strengths and shapes of your body's chewing parts that develop when they're used. When it comes to eating, there are mechanical nutrients involved as well as dietary ones. Unfortunately for us, it's become easier and easier to outsource our chewing—although it's unlikely we think of it that way.

From *The Human Machine* by George B. Bridgman:

> The mouth was made to cut and grind food. To save this trouble and work, mechanical devices such as the millstone were put into operation. Here the upper stone ground while the lower was stationary. In the human machine, the upper stone is fixed and the

> lower does the grinding. The only movable bone of the skull is the lower jaw [Author's note: More recent information reveals there are a lot of joints in the skull; ask any craniosacral therapist.] which hinges to the head just in front of the ear. It acts as a lever of the third order. The cutting and grinding force is controlled by powerful muscles. The one that raises the lower jaw is named the temporal muscle.

With the invention of the mill (and likely before), we began outsourcing our personal chewing work to other people who moved (in non-chewing ways) to build and operate the mills. To the list of inventions that mechanically break down food so we don't have to use our teeth and jaw, you can also add: blender, grinder, knives, food processer, grater, meat tenderizers, and your stove and oven. Forget, for a moment, all those *other* outsourced whole-body movements by which one turns plants and animals into something edible; at this point I'm only speaking of the work that used to be done by our own faces, that final step in which food becomes, literally, edible.

It's come on slowly, but as we humans have created technologies to make eating less work, we've changed our shape to match. Like an excellent autobiography, the story of our habits is stored in our skeletons, to be read by those in the future. Similarly, bones left behind by certain groups of people reveal that some (not unlike many of us today) have teeth that didn't fit inside their jaw. This was the result of a non-hunter-gatherer diet,[1] a jaw shape stimulated (or not) by soft foods as well as not needing to use the teeth and jaw in lieu of tools to cut and process foods and hides.[2] This too-big-teeth/too-small-jaw issue is solely chalked up to evolutionary changes, but really it's difficult to separate someone's mechanical environment from their genes. Before you conclude that particular changes are brought about by evolution, you have to consider how a lifetime of movement can influence the size and shape of a body.

It turns out that if you give a group of the same animal different diets, the jaw (and other face bones) will grow differently, their bone shapes reflecting their diet. If your diet is more challenging to chew, you'll grow a more robust structure to chew with.[3]

According to Bridgman, the mill has been saving us trouble and work, but I ask: Has it, really? If part of what the jaw, teeth, and face bones require as inputs to develop and maintain their structures—which are integral to basic biological functions like chewing—is eliminated, you must then figure out how to get that input elsewhere, or treat any symptoms that arise in the case of a (mechanical) nutrient deficiency. We don't talk much about orthodontia being an entire field of study dedicated to a symptom of outsourced movement, or consider the efforts spent on trips to the orthodontist, or wonder where all that hardware and those tools come from. Who makes those? Under what conditions, using what materials (found or mined where and how and by whom?) and fuel (taken from what source?)? What about trips to the doctor, to figure out the pain (osteoarthritis) in the temporomandibular joint and the gadgets to put in our mouth at night, or to the bone specialist to figure out the osteoporosis in the jaw? And the trips to the pharmacy? All of which require a trip to the bank, if you know what I mean.

Many have begun thinking more deeply about nutrition, which

has prompted a return to a whole-food diet. Sort of. We're at the point of considering the dietary nutrients of food—the chemistry—but have yet to think of the mechanical nutrients brought about by whole food. We think of processed foods as those foods that have been altered chemically in some way, to preserve or change how that food occurred in nature. Thus, when we use the term "whole food," we're not really talking about physically intact, entire animals and plants as much as we are *chemically* intact food. But what if there is more than one type of processed food?

For example, this is a carrot.

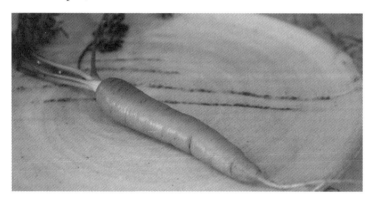

And this is a carrot.

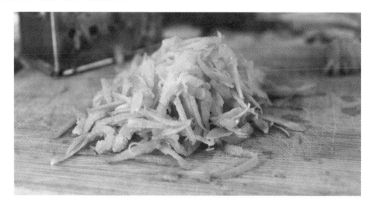

And this is a carrot.

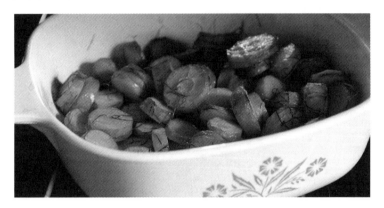

You'd probably consider all of these carrot versions a "whole" food, but they are not all the same; they are not all whole. While they could all be equal in *dietary* nutrients, each requires different work from your body and thus each contains different *mechanical* nutrients.

To be clear, I have nothing against processing and cooking food. I love food, I love all manner of traditionally processed "whole" foods. (And, P.S., there are even some non-traditionally processed foods I adore.) Our ability to process food has freed up time for us and enabled us to make big leaps forward in other areas. I appreciate my knives and blenders and mortars and pestles. My point is only that there is a benefit to, and perhaps even a need for, not *always* using them, if we want to be fully nourished.

1. von Cramon-Taubadel, N. 2011. "Global Human Mandibular Variation Reflects Differences in Agricultural and Hunter-Gatherer Subsistence strategies." *Proceedings of the National Academy of Sciences*. doi: 10.1073/pnas.1113050108.

2. Clement, A., Simon Hillson, Ignacio de la Torre, and Grant Townsend. 2008. "Tooth Use in Aboriginal Australia." *Archaeology International* 11: 37–40. doi. org/10.5334/ai.1111.

3. Lieberman, D. E., G. E. Krovitz, F. W. Yates, M. Devlin, and M. St. Claire. 2004. "Effects of Food Processing on Masticatory Strain and Craniofacial Growth in a Retrognathic Face." *Journal of Human Evolution* 46(6): 655–77.

Additional Sources

Zink, Katherine D. and Daniel E. Lieberman. 2016. "Impact of Meat and Lower Palaeolithic Food Processing Techniques on Chewing in Humans." *Nature* 531: 500–503. doi:10.1038/nature16990.

MAMMALS SUCK

There are all sorts of outsourced movements, some easier to see than others.

Imagine an apple. Then imagine all the things you can create from that apple: apple juice, grated apple, cooked apple, apple slices. Perhaps you could extract the pectin, or the vitamin C, or dehydrate the apple, grind it, and make apple powder. (I don't know if apple powder is an actual thing, but bear with me.)

Each of these is a derivative of an apple, but eating them is not the same as eating the apple they came from. To eat that apple is to be affected by both *what is contained in* and *what you experience by* eating the apple.

The forces created by chewing plants and animals have a purpose, meaning food has at least one purpose beyond providing dietary nutrients: Food provides the necessary mechanical stimulation for the development of multiple systems. I mentioned bone development in my previous essay because that's the variable I chose to consider, but chewing (and ripping and tearing and swallowing) movements and the frequency of these movements affect the function and future state of all tissues and actions involved: the jaw bone, the muscles of the face and throat, swallowing strength, vocal cord development, Eustachian tubes, sinuses, face muscles, the glands in the throat, and the list goes on. *All* tissues involved in eating are loaded differently when we've outsourced much of our mouth's work to various technologies.

Now imagine a milk-filled breast and the things you can create with it, like breast milk and dehydrated breast milk. Pendulous movement. A wet shirt.

Just as eating apple products provides different mechanical nutrients from those you would get when eating a whole apple, the experience of suckling milk from a breast differs, mechanically, from drinking that exact same breast milk from a bottle or a cup or sucking it out of a puddle on the ground.

Breastfeeding is a phenomenon often researched in modern hunter-gatherer populations to get a sense (or as close to a sense as possible) of how humans have fed their young historically. At first glance, breastfeeding seems costly from an ecological perspective.[4] As a lactating mom, you have to eat more, yet because you're usually carrying your kid on your body, you also move more slowly, meaning other people might have to gather a portion of the food you gathered before you were nursing, and perhaps your body has to do the extra work to store energy for your offspring, making you heavier, thus costing you more calories to move. The whole thing seems so work-intensive. But at the same time, breastfeeding can be efficient in that one doesn't need to forage newborn-friendly foods—your body converts what you eat into newborn food naturally. It comes stored right there in your body; you're not learning to deal with new containers. And then there's the fact that the act of breastfeeding does more than just provide dietary nutrients; it provides a particular mouth and jaw workout—mechanical nutrients—to the baby that the baby might not be able to get elsewhere. In this way, breastfeeding can be viewed as extremely efficient: alongside the nutrition it provides, it also offers a baby the acquisition of anatomy and skills necessary for biologically essential tasks in the future.

Baby mammals work hard to get milk out of the teat. Or, at least, baby human mammals do; I'm not sure about other animals. We say mammals suck, but what they really do is work their tongue and jaw hard to "milk" the breast. A baby's jaw bone moves up and down to compress and release the areola. The baby's tongue undulates—assuming numerous shapes, each working tongue muscles differently—similar to a farmer rolling their fist down a cow's teat. Other tongue muscles contract to curl the tongue around the nipple to channel the milk to the back of the throat to cue the swallowing reflex. Cycling changes in jaw and tongue position repeatedly change the shape of the face, and thereby these means increase and decrease the volume of the mouth to create a vacuum that draws out milk in a combination of milking and sucking—or suckling, as it's called. The nervous system coordinates the suckling, swallowing, and breathing so that all the essentials happen in concert.[5]

I'm exhausted just thinking about all the work that's involved, but here's the thing: breastfeeding is a mechanical feedback loop. Working for the milk is what, at least in part, keeps the milk coming.

As with all workouts, frequency and duration matter. Working out twice a day for thirty minutes is different from working out once for an hour. Working out for a year is different from working out for three. Similarly, each frequency and duration of breastfeeding should be considered a unique "movement program" as different scenarios alter the physical structure of a baby's mouth and face and all the parts involved in suckling differently.

When researching breastfeeding, one needs to note that "a breastfed child" could be defined as a child breastfed once or twice a day (even if they are drinking breast milk the rest of the day), a child who breastfeeds multiple times a day for thirty minutes at a time, or a child who breastfeeds a few times an hour for just a few minutes at a time. It could mean a child who breastfeeds for six months, or a year, or three years. My point being, we've been considering a partial nutrient profile when it comes to diet, and as more and more data is gathered regarding the role breast milk and breastfeeding play in the development of a human animal, we must delineate in a way that captures all the nutrients.

While many are still operating under the biological imperative of a species to propagate (a cold way of saying that we keep on making those cute and cuddly babies), we live in a time where the economic reality is that most of us have to work. Breastfeeding is easily, sometimes necessarily, and often reluctantly outsourced—in many cases adequate milk supply simply doesn't occur, for a variety of reasons that still need to be better researched and could easily occupy an entire book.

Alongside this practice of outsourcing (regardless of the reasons), has come mouths—and functions of and within the mouth (and the nose, and breathing)—that require many interventions to reclaim basic oral-motor functions like chewing, swallowing, and breathing; as well as speech therapies, dentistry, and orthodontics for tooth and jaw formation, not to mention non-mechanical therapies for nutritional and gut bacteria deficits.

A technology-rich culture can often mask the costs of a technology by creating new ones, in a cycle that repeats and repeats. This makes it seem like all our needs are met eventually, at no extra cost—but it's not that there are no costs so much as the costs are displaced. Imagine if businesses and insurance companies factored in the cost of all the seemingly inevitable therapies we receive throughout our lives that are necessary to restore basic biological function, as it calculated the cost of maternity leave? Imagine if the work necessary to breastfeed—the work of the child and the mother—was viewed as a calculated investment toward saving time and work in the future?

It's easier to choose to outsource movement when there are no clear solutions presented (i.e., the need to work is a reality and society is okay with the ramifications despite their unsustainability) and when the long-term costs to outsourcing—costs assumed later, by us, others, and the planet—are muddled or, worse, hidden away. Both are happening, and frankly, both suck.

---

4. Wander, K., and S. M. Mattison. 2013. "The Evolutionary Ecology of Early Weaning in Kilimanjaro, Tanzania." *Proceedings of the Royal Society B: Biological Sciences* 280(1768). doi:10.1098/rspb.2013.1359

5. Elad, David, Pavel Kozlovsky, Omry Blum et al. 2014. "Biomechanics of Milk Extraction During Breast-feeding." *PNAS* 111(14): 5230–5235. doi:10.1073/pnas.1319798111.

Additional Sources

Lamb, Michael E. 2005. *Hunter-Gatherer Childhoods: Evolutionary, Developmental & Cultural Perspectives.* New Jersey: Aldine Transaction.

Palmer, Brian, M.D. 1998. "The Influence of Breastfeeding on the Development of the Oral Cavity: A Commentary." *Journal of Human Lactation* 14(2): 93–98. <brianpalmerdds.com/bfeed_oralcavity.htm>

Also see this video: "Biomechanics of Milk Extraction During Breast-Feeding": youtu.be/bJg9mC0x34M.

For more on breastfeeding, including great resources for support, see Appendix 3.

FORAGE

Every day, in addition to the tasks required for work, are those must-dos on my list: spend time with my family, educate my children, source wholesome ingredients, feed my family, move my body, move my kids' bodies, and expose our bodies to nature (sunlight, the sounds of nature, temperature variations, etc.). Other to-dos vary day by day, but these are the ones that sit at the front of my mind all the time.

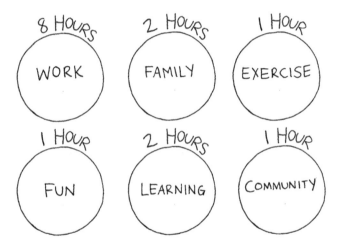

When I look at these to-dos as a list, I start calculating the time necessary to accomplish them all. I require *at least* a few hours of daily movement. I need to shop and cook, which takes a couple of hours as well. Playing games or reading books—designed with some learning schema for kids—can also take an hour to facilitate. Right away, each day, I'm overwhelmed because I do not have the six extra hours in the day to facilitate what I consider to be essential tasks alongside the reality that I must work. I'm also uncomfortable approaching the essentials from the perspective of "minimum time," because do I really want to figure out the *minimums* when it comes to spending time with family? No, I do not.

I used to think of my obligations in series. Each holding their own area, in seemingly unrelated rows, were all the categories of obligation I had to attend to: work (i.e., making money), parenting, relationships, household, work, community, movement, and work again.

Nature is a good teacher, and I have learned quite a bit about efficiency from observing it. In nature, functions aren't plotted side by side, each holding their own personal space in time. Nature accomplishes many tasks at the same time. With this in mind, I changed the way I thought about and scheduled my own life. Instead of breaking up my obligations and allotting time to each fractured component (i.e., twenty minutes to get food, forty-five minutes for some exercise, an hour to spend with my kids, four hours to produce something work-related), I organized my life essentials so that the same portion of time fulfills multiple obligations. I call this way of relating time to essential tasks "stacking your life."

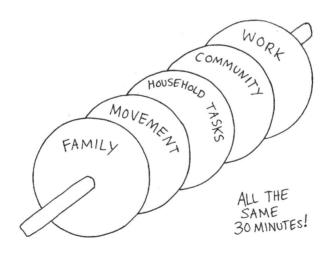

Arranging your life to accomplish multiple things simultaneously is not new—it's often called multitasking. Stacking your life and multitasking are similar in many ways, but they're different in at least one fundamental way: Stacking your life often requires that you change the way you're currently meeting a need. Looking for an approach or activity that meets multiple goals is critical to stacking your life, and is different from trying to fit all the things you're currently trying to do into the same piece of time.

For example, foraging with my family was one way I found I could regularly meet all of my obligations—to myself, my family, my community, my planet—and it was an activity I had never considered as a "solution" until I tried it.

In addition to meeting my more tangible obligations to others (feeding my kids), foraging allows me to meet my needs of behaving in real life in a way that aligns with who I want to be on paper. The natural by-product of foraging and not outsourcing this work to other people and companies is that I'm accomplishing my must-dos and not trying to schedule them as separate events.

I am like a small child in my foraging skills, but like a child, I am persistent in my learning. When I first became a parent, I created foraging scenarios for our family. I'd say something like, "We need to go out and find some food," and I steered the kids toward some plant/tree/patch a quarter of a mile away. Along the way we would crawl up and down ditches, climb trees, and stop to pee. (We always need to pee about ninety seconds after leaving the house.)

On one particular trip, a neighbor greeted the kids, who told him we were going food hunting. He donated to our cause and gave us some extra food from his garden we then needed to carry. Later we arrived at our destination and gathered, which included finding and operating sticks to knock fruit down, jumping to grab and wobble limbs, and bending and squatting to gather our bounty.

It wasn't a quick walk to the tree and back (as those of you with kids can imagine); it was a two-hour event. YES, *two hours* to walk half a mile. But before you go thinking, "I don't have two hours of free time, so this doesn't apply to me," let me remind you of my earlier list. In this instance, I moved for two hours; I was outside for two hours; I was with my family for two hours; I was offline and screen-free for two hours; I fed my family, or more importantly, *they fed themselves*; my kids moved outside for two hours; my kids learned for two hours, all the stuff I want to "teach" them about nature, healthy eating, where food comes from, how to use their bodies, personal responsibility, wastefulness, and consumerism. It was all covered in a foraging session and I didn't have to say a word; it was learning in its most natural form. The way I see it, it *only* took two hours for what I had previously figured to take six or ten.

These days, these same kids, with their ever-expanding knowledge of plants garnered from their nature school, teach their parents, in a role reversal that is empowering for them and inspiring to me.

Stacking functions is not a new idea. Permaculture enthusiasts have long been stacking agricultural functions in a way that lets nature do its efficient work. What I propose here is that we need to think of movement in the same way. To keep our movement functions sustainable—ensuring that we and other humans are able to move both now and in the future—we need to adopt a practice of movement permaculture. Foraging can be an easy, fun-filled first step to a sustainable and "stacked" life.

If you're looking for the nuts and bolts—and seeds and tubers—of how to get started foraging, please see Appendix 2.

KITCHEN MOVEMENT

Although we've been able to outsource the work necessary to meet some of our biological needs, we haven't been able to outsource all of it. Because humans evolved performing the same general movements at the same general frequencies for thousands of years, and because these movements are part of what determines and maintains our structure, these general, traditional movements could be considered an essential part of our anatomy, in that our bodies would be different without them.

Movement is a renewable resource, but unlike other commodities, it renews through use; your future movement is made possible by movements you're doing today. And so, as we spend less and less of our movement on our personal food consumption, we are essentially spending tomorrow's movement on the luxury of being still today. In five, ten, or twenty years, if you decide you want to start moving more for your health or happiness, you may find that your knees no longer feel good when you climb hills, that your hips creak and protest when you walk, that your feet can't support you without increasingly structured shoes.

And even if you've spent your food-procuring movement on non-food movements, someone, somewhere, is doing the movements necessary to make your food, or fueling the machines that do the work, or cutting the forests or mining the earth to make the machines or the fuel. The privilege of being able to outsource essential movements for preferred ones creates a burden on others and on the planet. We've been told we can vote with our dollars to support more ethical business practices, but what if we also performed simple movements to consume less overall? When you

FORCED CHILD LABOR: DO YOU KNOW WHERE THAT CAME FROM?

It's become second nature to many of us to check out the business practices of the companies we buy from—what their labor conditions are, where their products are made—but it's still pretty new (to me, at least) to consider where even the most perceived-as-ethical companies obtain their raw materials.

A couple of years ago I stumbled on an article about the child slavery involved in producing the cocoa used in the various chocolate candies I grew up with. I didn't quite believe the article—I couldn't imagine that I was only just hearing this information, or that products blatantly made in part by child slaves would be on our grocery store shelves. So I began an investigation that led me to a website created by the US Department of Labor. This page contains resources that list which countries produce which goods via forced (slave) labor, child labor, and forced child labor. I encourage you to investigate the page on your own, if only to become aware of the issues at hand. The Bureau of International Labor Affairs has also created a "Sweat and Toil" smartphone app that can tell you which goods are known to be manufactured via morally questionable practices (useful to check when you're shopping, especially for chocolate, and ordering your favorite beverage, especially if it's coffee).

While you're downloading that app to your phone, I also suggest you google "conflict minerals Congo" to learn more about the role that your smartphone is playing in these matters.

Visit the Bureau of International Labor Affairs website here: dol. gov/agencies/ilab/resources/reports/child-labor

App: Sweat and Toil: Child Labor, Forced Labor, and Human Trafficking Around the World by the U.S. Department of Labor

Further reading: *Blood and Earth: Modern Slavery, Ecocide, and the Secret to Saving the World*, by Kevin Bales. (Or start with his interview here: npr.org/sections/goatsand-soda/2016/01/20/463600820/todays-slaves-often-work-for-enterprises-that-destroy-the-environment)

move your body more, directly for your food, it not only serves your own body but also makes you, personally, less of a contributor to the problems of unnecessary oil consumption, slave labor, mistreatment of farm workers, production of unnecessary items, and the destruction of the planet.

Our historical outsourcing of movement over and over again for hundreds of years has led us to where we are right now with respect to the amount of movement you and I need to do in order to eat. Where once we spent hours each day exchanging the movements involved in walking, running, bending, squatting, carrying, pounding, rubbing, lifting, digging, and mashing for a day's worth of calories, we spend almost no movement (and lots of money on fuel) to drive to a store and wander the aisles to buy overly packaged food—foraged, planted, picked, dug, processed, and flown or driven there by other people.

One could argue that movement for food is no longer essential, but I guess that depends on your definition of essential. You have an eating requirement, you have a movement requirement, and you have a requirement not to place copious work on others in your tribe if you want that tribe to succeed—after all, their success is also yours. You have a need, one could say, to pull your own weight when it comes to food.

I'm not saying you have to give up your coconut flour and almond milk, but what if you looked at engaging with your food mechanically as a way to not only increase your movement but also decrease your reliance on electricity or the food industry, even if only in a small way? You can grow some of your own food (it's hard to be still in a garden) or forage, even just a tiny bit. Buying nuts in their shells and spending an hour or so sitting on the ground (or squatting) to crack them open with rocks is a movement-filled lesson in "how food grows" for little ones.

Swap out one electrical device for an old-fashioned equivalent where no electricity is needed! Not because you're a Luddite, but because you've listed "move more" and "consume less fossil fuel" as goals. (Somebody's grandmother used to beat egg whites into a meringue *with a fork*. You gonna get whipped by somebody's grandmother *because your arms get too tired*?)

Walk to your local grocery store (do I have to say "bring your own bags"?) or learn how to butcher your own meat, make your own jerky, fruit leather, wine, beer, or bread. Pick your own vegetables. Lay your own eggs.

Just kidding about the eggs.

Or you can do none of these things. Simply learning to recognize your own choices in the matter and to see how you relate to the bigger picture can be impactful. Awareness, after all, is its own nutrient.

A SEDENTARY CULTURE EATS

I often write about the physical weaknesses that persist in a sedentary culture and also how many of those weaknesses are part of a reduction in necessary biological functions and are normalized and/or explained by things other than a lack of movement.

The *Washington Post* published an article[6] highlighting a pilot and follow-up study on how American kids are throwing away the apples given to them for lunch. As it turns out, they throw the whole fruit away because eating it is too much work. Slice it, and they'll eat it.

According to the article, "A child holding a whole apple has to break the skin, eat around the core, and deal with the hassle of holding a large fruit," and older girls in particular found whole fruits messy and unattractive to eat.[7]

In 2014 Americans ate 511 million sliced apples, and this statistic is driving the food industry to focus their attention on pre-sliced, treated, and packaged apples. If we're considering only dietary nutritional value here, then "at least they're eating apples, and that's good, right?" applies. But if we broaden our scope to an ecological perspective, we'll see that the cost of our children not being practiced or strong enough to eat a whole food includes the work necessary to slice and often package the food (typically with plastic).

This is why I find it increasingly relevant to consider movement from an ecological perspective. Without framing our movement habits relative to the world, it's easy to miss the cost of outsourcing work necessary to meet our own biological needs. *Our children are too weak to eat whole apples; they were not provided with an environment necessary to develop strong chewing skills; and now other humans and the planet are burdened by their unnecessary weakness.* This is a matter of movement and is also why movement matters.

---

6. Ferdman, Roberto A. 2016. "A Clever Tweak to How Apples Are Being Sold is Making Everyone Eat More of Them." *Washington Post*, May 19. <washingtonpost.com/news/wonk/wp/2016/05/19/the-apple-industrys-strange-savior/>

7. Wansink, Brian, David R. Just, Andrew S. Hanks, and Laura E. Smith. 2013. "Pre-Sliced Fruit in School Cafeterias." *American Journal of Preventative Medicine* 44(5): 477-48.

MOVEMENT AS A COMMODITY

Movement is a commodity, once exchanged directly for food. Throughout the human timeline, barring a major environmental shift, an adult could eat as much as their (and their tribe's) movement skill provided, and in this way there was a balance of movement and food.

Food is naturally the fuel for movement, and movement the fuel for food acquisition. But at some point, individuals began outsourcing food-related movements to others willing to do them in exchange for non–biologically essential but equally appealing commodities, thus forming, I would suggest, the backbone of currency as we use it today.

Freedom from food-related movements afforded the opportunity for some to move their bodies in production of other things, and over a relatively short period of time (the last two hundred thousand years, but most accelerated over the last few hundred), most humans went from having days filled with a wide range of general, survival-related movements to spending their days on more specialized labor-intensive skills. As time passed, machines were built to assume many of the physical movements necessary for production—food or otherwise—and many were left with jobs operating machines or being part of the management (directly or indirectly) of other individuals still doing copious amounts of a few specialized movements on behalf of many.

Today, most humans can be divided into two "movement specialist" groups (meaning, groups of specialized movers). First, there are those humans—paid and forced/slave laborers—who spend the bulk of their lives laboring for items to benefit others.

They do so by performing a narrow range of highly repetitive movements that leave them overtaxed in some movements and poorly nourished in others. Second, there are those humans who are rich in movement-free time, because their food and other products are, thanks to our economic systems, brought to them by the movements performed by the first group. This second group spend the bulk of their movement-free time being sedentary and allot only a small portion of time (if any) to specialized movements necessary for sport and exercise programs, or work with their bodies to perform very specific tasks (e.g., builders, dancers, professional athletes). Either way, their movements rarely cover the full range of motions they need and would be getting if they were moving in order to feed themselves directly. So like the first group, to whom they have outsourced much of their daily movements, they also suffer from poor movement nutrition. There are almost no remaining "movement generalists" who are meeting all their movement nutrient needs, as only a few clusters of humans continue to hunt and gather for their food and survival.

Unfortunately for the last of the movement generalists, and all of us, ultimately, we've propped our technologies up on the globe's wilderness, and take little issue with spending hunter-gatherers' habitat "over there" on our stillness here—likely because we're not aware of the role we each play, individually, via personal outsourced movement.

While many people support a conservation ideal on paper, and grasp the concept that wilderness is finite and that our habits are wilderness-expensive, our daily actions suggest we either don't truly perceive the cost and unsustainability of our lifestyle, or we are simply unsure of how to begin to live in a different way.

Because we all still eat, movements relating to food acquisition can be an easy portal through which we can each reclaim some of the movement we've outsourced to others. You can improve the movement nutrition of your food at the macro or micro level, depending on what is feasible for you. You can walk to your local market instead of driving. You can shop for seasonal food and for local ingredients that took less fossil fuel to get to market, foods that were labored for by people whose working conditions you are fully aware of. You can raise your own proteins (eggs, small or large animals, legumes) and grow a garden. You can choose less-processed foods and physically work the ingredients yourself. You can build your meals around simple foods that need to be chewed. At whatever level you approach spending your movement on food, the physical burden of feeding you will be more greatly assumed by you, thus your food will nourish you more fully and tax others and the earth less. I believe this is called a win-win.

DEAR KATY

Q I HAVE CERTAIN PHYSICAL DISABILITIES THAT PREVENT ME FROM WALKING, LET ALONE FORAGING FOR FOOD. IS THERE ANY WAY FOR ME TO "STACK MY LIFE" WHEN IT COMES TO FOOD?

A Certainly! "Stacking your life" often has to do with finding another way to meet a need you're currently meeting in a way that's not serving as many aspects of your life as you'd like. Many of us like the foods we like or are used to, and don't often think about the journey our food has taken to arrive on our plate. You could likely make significant headway reducing the outsourced movement of your life simply by buying foods grown close to where you live. This could mean shopping at farmers' markets (or, if there isn't one physically accessible to you, having a CSA box delivered) or choosing seasonally appropriate foods (i.e., squashes in the fall, berries in the summer) so that you're not selecting foods that have been grown and flown in from other parts of the globe. There is a physical strength necessary to overcome food "wants" or cravings and I can tell you from experience that retraining your palate is not easy, but it is practical and hugely impactful! Make a list of the foods you purchase weekly and do a little research to get informed on the growing and harvesting practices of these items (for example, the chocolate industry is notorious for using human trafficking and child slave labor). Choose to buy brands that only source their ingredients in a way that aligns with your beliefs, or shift your taste preferences for foods that occur locally (to whatever degree you define this). In this way, you are stacking your life by participating in activism and helping the global community as well as your local food producers, while also doing the biologically necessary work of feeding yourself.

In the same way I point out that movement is bigger than exercise, I want to emphasize that movement is bigger than the movements of our own bodies. The movement of food towards our house matters too, because it's made up of the movement of other people's bodies and parts that make up the natural world.

And one more stacking note: If you have a place to eat outside, you're also stacking your life by reducing need for heating/air conditioning/lighting as well as getting doses of movement in the form of regulating your body temperature, looking to a distance, and letting natural noise bend the sensors in your ears—all at the same time as you picnic. If you do it with friends, you're building community too. Stack away!

Q I'VE HEARD YOU TALK AND HAVE SEEN YOUR WRITING ABOUT THE VARIOUS WAYS YOU'VE "STACKED YOUR LIFE" BY DOING SOME OF YOUR WORK (E.G., TAKING PHONE CALLS ON HIKES) IN NATURE. MY TIME SPENT IN NATURE IS PRECIOUS AND THERE'S NO WAY I'M BRINGING MY WORK INTO THE WOODS WITH ME. WHERE CAN I GO FROM HERE?

A I wouldn't suggest anyone muddle already established nature time with technology or work. Keep that time as it is. My suggestion is that you "nature up" your work time by looking to see where it's possible to remove some of the physical constraints that come with the time you've allotted to "work" or productivity. My recommendation isn't that you take work-related phone calls on your hike, but rather that you set out on foot to do your calls. It's a subtle difference that has more to do with scheduling and intention than it does with the motions of your arms and legs. If you can get in a headspace that allows you to see the bulk of what you do for work doesn't have to be done sitting at your desk or inside an office, I believe you'll find abundant time and space *just sitting there* that could be used to nourish your body better while you continue to be productive—without any need to encroach on the time you've set aside to fully engage with nature.

Q   MY LEAST FAVORITE WORD IS "WHATEVER," WHEN IT'S USED TO CONCLUDE A SENTENCE. I'M FRUSTRATED BY ITS USE BECAUSE IT SEEMS THE USER WON'T EXPEND THEIR ENERGY TO CLARIFY AND STATE THE IDEAS THAT THEY'VE ATTEMPTED TO COMMUNICATE. I'M WONDERING, DO YOU HAVE A LEAST FAVORITE WORD OR PHRASE?

A   Currently, my least favorite phrase is "the real world," when used to explain why a habit or change can't be made. For instance, "I'd like to move more and work less and grow a garden and give up products that come by labor and plane from the other side of the planet, *but I live in the real world.*"

The thing is, so does everyone and everything else. When

someone uses the phrase "the real world," they're implying, iron-ically, the opposite of the truly diverse, possibility-filled real world. Maybe they feel their family or community or culture they participate in won't support them making changes to their lifestyle, but it's critical to recognize that they've defined "the real world" to be their personal experience, or the "real to them" world. Their experience matters and is part of the real world, of course, but that's true of everyone else's experience, including those who've made those supposedly unrealistic changes. An alternative to "I live in the real world" could be "I'd like to move more and work less and grow a garden and give up products that come by labor and plane from the other side of the planet, *but I can't see how that's possible for me.*" It's much more feasible to bring about change when we see the issue is with ourselves, and not a problem of the solution not existing in the universe.

just move

Never does nature say one thing and wisdom
another.

—JUVENAL

While movement has been around since the beginning of
time, exercise is a human construct in its infancy. All exercise is movement, of course, but not all movement is exercise. By
this I mean there are numerous movements we perform and could
perform each day that do not fall into the clinical definition of
exercise (physical activity that is planned, structured, and repetitive and that has a final or an intermediate objective to improve or
maintain physical fitness), or even our personal understanding of
physical activity that is beneficial to our body. For example, breastfeeding is a movement that, like exercise, brings about a certain
strength profile and shape to the mover's body, but breastfeeding
wouldn't fit into most people's current definition of "exercise for
health"—it's just what babies have historically needed to do to
survive.

One of the characteristics of exercise is that it's performed
solely for the purpose of reaping physiological benefits (physical

conditioning), whereas the goal of non-exercise movement is to reap the non-movement benefits of physical activity.

Going for a one-mile or thirty-minute walk to strengthen your legs, burn some calories, and stretch your muscles is an example of exercise. Walking a mile to the store because you need to pick up something for dinner is an example of movement. Both may use certain muscles within the body in exactly the same way, but there is a big-picture difference regarding how biological needs—of the moving human, of other humans, and of the environment—are being met and which costs are being accrued during that period of time. And so by "all exercise is movement, but not all movement is exercise," I also mean that there is a difference in the outcome between a human moving and a human exercising that you might not see until you assess the impact of that movement outside of the individual physical adaptations to each scenario.

There is a tremendous interest in human movement as a solution to many modern ailments, and we have a lot of data on how exercise positively impacts health and many physiological variables. However, we have yet to contemplate what a sustainable model of human movement is beyond the recommended handful of hours a week we've predetermined people should exercise-for-health. We've reduced movement to such miniscule levels within our daily lives that it's no wonder we don't even contemplate how our movement—or, more specifically, our lack of it—counts in a global context. Human behavior is rarely incorporated into ecological models, except in very specific circumstances, such as visitor impact on national parks or in models of climate change. Many humans are hyperconsumers, engaging in behavior that could be measured by a human's carbon footprint. But our individual carbon footprints, certainly the portion necessary for essentials, could also be viewed more as a symptom of sedentarism—consumption brought about by a lack of movement or ability to move.

Pleading for the reduced use of technologies (like a car or heat and air conditioning in our home) that we require to compensate for our weaknesses is an inefficient pursuit if we need these technologies to move on our behalf. A more direct approach is for each of us to demonstrate how we would require less carbon to fuel our movement through pursuit of greater movement and strength— something a vast majority of people would agree they want more of anyway. Yes, many will need to eat more once they start moving more, but because movement is also a necessity, the increase in caloric consumption can be thought of as an investment that, in the future, reduces your need for technologies like medicine and surgical interventions used to treat issues stemming from local or whole-body sedentarism. Also, the more you choose wild foods and local foods, the less carbon you "spend" on eating (i.e., not all foods cost the same in terms of production).

We've yet to investigate how a specific human behavior, such as our lack of movement, impacts an ecosystem,[1] let alone how a single human's whole-life behavior affects it, because it makes the model very complicated. However, we should not avoid complexity because of the challenge it presents; that's why they call it scientific *rigor*. And we definitely don't want to avoid adding more parts just because we might not like what that shows us about the lifestyle we have grown accustomed to.

Research could begin with quantification of the carbon use

necessary to live the average day of the average sedentary person (which is almost all of us). We could calculate the energy used to eat, maintain a comfortable-to-us temperature, to transport us—the fundamental technologies most of us use each day to meet our basic needs. The good news is, we do not have to wait for proof that we are consuming more than we need to. What research says or has yet to say on the matter doesn't determine the status of the ecosystem; it merely reports it. You yourself can quantify the movements you could be doing that you don't or can't, and the resources you require to continue outsourcing movement and then literally take action. Science does not, nor can it, dole out personal responsibility. You, yourself, have to decide to move through your life in a way that supports your own physiology and doesn't unnecessarily encroach on the movement of all others things in the world. You, yourself, must get moving.

---

1. Alberti, Marina, John M. Marzluff, Eric Shulenberger, Gordon Bradley, Clare Ryan, and Craig Zumbrunnen. 2003. "Integrating Humans into Ecology: Opportunities and Challenges for Studying Urban Ecosystems." *BioScience* 53(12): 1169-1179, doi:10.1641/0006-3568(2003)053[1169:IHIEOA]2.0.CO;2

PART-MINDED

Science is the pursuit of understanding the phenomena of the natural world. Because phenomena are complex, the scientific method is used to break down each phenomenon into a series of smaller parts to study separately, the intent being that if we can understand the parts more deeply, we will then know the phenomenon. The breaking down of a phenomenon into parts is called reduction, but you could also call reduction an unpacking or *unstacking* of a phenomenon.

To research a part, we often have to separate it from its natural state. There is not another way science can be done; still, reduction has repercussions. The act of separating changes what we see and affects the conclusions we come to. For example, anatomists have been studying the brain by removing its membranous casing. And those who have studied the membranes exclusively used a particular cutting method to create the membrane samples they wanted to look at. Each of these researchers were, it turned out, obliterating the brain's lymphatic vessels in the process, leading scientists to the conclusion that the brain didn't *have* a lymphatic system and was immune-privileged (meaning that antigens—foreign substances that make your body create antibodies—could enter the brain without inducing an inflammatory immune response). But it turns out that the brain *does* have a lymphatic system,[2] which was discovered when one lab used a new method to slice out the brain part they wanted to study.

And then there are trees. Most of us know some things about how trees work. The roots of a tree anchor it to the ground, and uptake water and minerals for the tree. The trunk grows to the best height for the tree, and serves as a nutrient highway, bringing the minerals from the ground to the leaves and taking the tree's food (carbohydrates), created in the leaves via photosynthesis, back down toward the roots.

But the parts of a working, living tree aren't just those listed above; the components of a working tree also include minerals, soil, sunlight, air. And here are some parts of a working tree that we've only just discovered: other trees. Yes, it appears trees use and assist other trees. This is different from the already observed passive inter- actions between trees, like other trees blocking sunlight or shaping wind patterns that eventually affect the growth, shape, and thus performance of a tree within the same area. Trees appear to actively work and communicate with each other:[3] older trees shunt nutri- ents to young trees as they're growing (and younger, smaller trees can send nutrients to bigger and older ones too); they (and other plants) send "I'm being attacked" messages to other trees that help those other trees prepare for an attack themselves,[4] and a tree of one species can share resources with a tree of another species at the time of year when it is flourishing, and the recipient will recipro- cate. But it turns out that other trees are not the only parts of a tree outside its own anatomy—you also need a fungus.

Mycorrhiza is a mutualistic symbiosis between a fungus and the roots of a plant. The plant nourishes the fungus and the fungus returns the favor, and in the last few years it's been observed that just as the air transports words from human to human, the fungus in a mycorrhiza transports signals tree to tree via a complex network. This means that all the parts making up a tree flourishing in nature aren't even contained within a tree—that the natural state of a working tree involves *treeothers*, as well as an entirely different species (the fungus).

While the reductive process in making scientific progress is imperfect, I cannot see another way that science can be done. We would not have had all of this scientific evidence about how trees and brains work if we hadn't had the part-by-part process. However, the information that comes from this unstacking process often gives us only a series of facts. It is the restacking and assembling of these individual facts, gathered from many different sciences, that enables us to gain insights into natural phenomena (i.e., the purpose of science). In other words, the other half of science—the partner to breaking nature down—is considering all the facts together. Unfortunately, we're often poorest at integrating the facts, and we are living at a time when an understanding of an intact nature has never been more critical. If we weren't living an unstacked life, and if we were more aware, generally, that our scientifically dissected parts aren't always drawing us a picture of the whole, would we have thought to look more broadly and learned about the function of mycorrhizae sooner?

We must stay aware that the whole is often greater than the sum of its isolated and studied parts. We cannot live on vitamins and other individual nutrients (e.g., proteins, carbohydrates, fats) extracted or separated from food; we need to eat numerous types of real, whole foods. Similarly, basing recommendations for what humans need to live a healthy life on knowledge of a few parts (to be clear, our knowledge even of nature-parts is grossly incomplete at this point) is leaving us poorly nourished in many areas.

I am not saying a part-by-part progression isn't necessary for scientific investigation, but rather, science's need for parts should not be mistaken for a human's need for parts. Humans don't require the parts; humans require the whole. Thus, in order to truly understand what we might require, we need to take into consideration not only a series of facts gathered by the practice of modern scientific investigation, but also the total body of knowledge and experience that has developed across all human societies through our evolutionary history—our collective human wisdom, if you like.

It seems to me that our part-by-part mentality, and perhaps even the need for science—the need to understand nature—has evolved as we've migrated out of a natural ecosystem. Our desire to understand nature scientifically came at the point when, from a lack of exposure, we no longer understood it through experience.

Many groups of people have (and many more used to have) knowledge of plants and their medicinal qualities, which foods to eat and when they are available, and how to process foods so the inedible becomes edible—all without possessing facts made available via a microscope. Human animals have understood natural phenomena well enough to thrive as a part of nature for millennia,[5] using this traditional knowledge to locate nutrient-dense food sources, get adequate movement, develop plant medicine, and fashion clothes and footwear, watercraft and weaponry. But these humans didn't only possess a traditional knowledge of nature; they were also skillful in the application of it. Their knowledge of natural food and movement wasn't separate from their skills in applying it.

The phenomenon of human movement has been recently separated from its natural context, in practice and in research. We're at the beginning of an understanding regarding movement. We have yet to consider how it works locally within the body, and how human movement facilitates necessary actions between human animals and between humans and other species. Uncoincidentally, the beginning of our pursuit of scientific knowledge regarding human movement comes at the end of our practice of regular movement—I'd suggest a group of humans has never before been this sedentary and survived. We have no idea how to move, and so we're turning to science to show us. (P.S. That's not science's role at all, but when you have an elder-free society, you have to turn to somewhere, and scientific data is where many of us are turning.) I do think science will eventually give us a list that we can reintegrate into a picture of how to move, but frankly, I don't think we have that long. Meaning, our scientific pursuits are made possible by sedentarism. We may run out of the natural resources we use to sustain ourselves without moving before science can tell us how to move in order to sustain ourselves.

So, my friends: Just as we don't need to know which nutrients are in food to know that we need to eat, we don't have to wait until science has parsed out more parts of the understanding of movement to know that we must move in order to survive. While the understanding of movement can definitely assist us in our transition from non-mover to mover, our physiology doesn't *require* the explanation, and we certainly don't require permission. We simply require movement.

---

2. Dissing-Olesen, Lasse, Soyon Hong, and Beth Stevens. 2015. "New Brain Lymphatic Vessels Drain Old Concepts." *EBioMedicine* 2(8): 776–777. PMC.

3. Gorzelak, M. A., A. K. Asay, B. J. Pickles, and S. W. Simard. 2015. "Inter-Plant Communication through Mycorrhizal Networks Mediates Complex Adaptive Behaviour in Plant Communities." *AoB Plants* 7: plv050.

4. Karban, Richard, Louie H. Yang, and Kyle F. Edwards. 2013. "Volatile Communication between Plants that Affects Herbivory: A Meta-Analysis." *Ecology Letters* 17: 44–52.

5. Mazzocchi, Fulvio. 2006. "Western Science and Traditional Knowledge: Despite Their Variations, Different Forms of Knowledge Can Learn from Each Other." *EMBO Reports* 7(5): 463–466. doi.org/10.1038/sj.embor.7400693.

STACK YOUR LIFE

I aspire to achieve the efficiency of a worker honeybee. A worker honeybee has one of those jobs with all-day movement packaged in. Its home is totally eco-friendly—easily repairable and entirely biodegradable, with each room *the perfect size.*[6] Its community is rocking—honeybees work together collectively to support the entire hive, a process that includes establishing a home, generating offspring, providing childcare, and putting up preserves for the winter. Nature isn't always benign (especially to the young virgin queens being hunted and killed by other young virgin queens), but it is efficient. No essential task in a honeybee's life occurs in isolation. The work necessary to meet its personal needs for food and movement and to perform its particular job on behalf of its community are happening simultaneously.

In fact, everything in what we call nature is happening at once. Which means the only thing organized unnaturally is that which we don't consider to be nature—*humanstuff.* We've carved ourselves away from nature, literally and in the way we talk about it. And perhaps because we are parsed, we parse nature, extracting parts of a phenomenon for investigative purposes to better understand nature. But regularly reducing everything from its natural state, ourselves included, has, I propose, influenced the way we think about how things work—including how *we* work, both physiologically and simply in terms of how we live over the course of a day.

My father, now eighty-nine years old, once told me the secret to life: don't multitask. I didn't get it. I was busy as a worker bee. And frankly, as a full-time self-employed mother of two, barely fitting in 48 percent of my "must-do-daily" tasks by doing two to four things at a time, the idea of no longer multitasking was paralyzing. There was no possible way for me to do everything I needed to do without doing multiple things at once. But what I've since come to realize is that while there is no possible way of doing everything I need to do without doing multiple things at once, the things I had been choosing to do at once weren't the best way of meeting my needs. So I propose the real secret to life (and I mean this literally, as in how to make life sustainable in the big picture): We've got to get inspired by the efficiency of the honeybees and start stacking.

Your current categories of obligation are likely similar to mine. You probably have to work, attend to your family, nurture a partnership and/or friendships, move, eat, drink, and be merry. Similarly, each of the people in your personal ecosystem (those in your home and close community—or hive, if you will) have their own categories of obligation that must be filled, which oftentimes involve your participation.

You've probably long since decided on the tasks you regularly use to meet all your categories of obligation, and I'd bet those tasks probably only ever address one or two obligations at a time. Meaning, the tasks you've selected force you to either allot only a small fraction of time and attention to what you've chosen to do—half an hour to cook supper, an hour at the gym, then a half hour with the kids before bed, etc.—or to sacrifice entire categories of need altogether (I'm thinking of someone preparing all the food from scratch for everyone in the family, but then having no time to go out for a hike, hang out with their community, or build their dream business). In either case, any lifestyle in which your biological needs are not all being met isn't working for you and the solution might be simpler than you think.

Like multitasking, stacking your life means using the same period of time to fulfill different functions, as I describe in the essay "Forage" on page 104. There are big differences between the two concepts, however, and they're not semantic; stacking your life and multitasking differ in how you approach meeting your various needs. Multitasking involves trying to accomplish many discrete tasks at once. Stacking your life involves the search for fewer tasks that meet multiple needs, which often requires that you're clear on what your needs actually are. Once you identify your needs and which tasks best serve you, you can attend to, pay attention to, get involved in, and focus upon a single task at hand that serves multiple obligations. Pretty sweet, right?

Which brings me back to the worker bee and its busy-ness and how I used to think. Back when I was feeling as busy as one, I imagined the worker bee's to-do list was similar in structure to mine: It worked—pollinated—the bulk of each day, and around that it had to fit in meals, get exercise, maintain its home and relationships, and tend to and bring home the bee-bacon for its young. It needed to move and also it needed to rest.

I was wrong, of course. A worker honeybee doesn't see itself as a pollinator and wake to pollinate; a worker honeybee wakes to get food. Driven by its biology and facilitated by its environment, its body is moved by the search, and parts of its anatomy passively collect and distribute pollen along the way, thus perpetuating its own food source in the future while meeting its own nutritional needs.

I could say that honeybees expertly stack their functions, and that all plants and animals expertly stack their functions, but here's the thing: Nothing in nature is stacking its functions. "Stacking functions" is a human construct that simply means trying to get back to how we work when we are in nature for the sake of efficiency when it comes to meeting our natural needs. *All of them*. It's the slow reverse-engineering of a modern world back to nature; it's recognizing that work is natural, but jobs are not. The type of work a bee does not only benefits itself but also its colony, the plants it pollinates, and those that utilize parts of plants for their own existence (which is most other animals). If a bee didn't need to gather its own nectar, if nectar were available right there within the bee's home, the work it performed would also cease to occur, and the side effects of a bee not moving for its food would impact more than its physical fitness; it would impact the ability of all other living things to survive.

Becoming as efficient as a bee by choosing to do work that reintegrates all the compartments of your life to better meet your personal needs, as well as the tasks necessary for your role in your community and in the world, requires a movement of your thoughts. Thinking differently is a process not so distinct from learning to move your arm or leg in a particular way to get a muscle to grow; your thoughts shape your choices. I believe we can exist in harmony with the earth, and all other things on it, once we have a firm understanding of our biological requirements (and no, they're not the technologies that have been developed to compensate when we fail to meet them). Once we observe that we can, in fact, meet our needs holistically rather than separately—by doing the work necessary for our own and our hive's survival—we'll be taxing the world less.

Stacking your life doesn't require the frantic pace and constant juggling of multitasking (thanks, Dad; you were right), but it does take awareness, community, and work—both mental and physical. The good news is that "get more awareness, a robust community, and increased physical and mental strength" were probably on your to-do list anyhow, so you're nailing this stack-your-life thing right out of the gate.

---

6. Hales, T. C. 1999. "The Honeycomb Conjecture." Cornell University Library. <arxiv.org/abs/math.MG/9906042>

MAXIMALISM

Tiny houses. Minimal footwear. That bestselling book from Marie Kondo, *The Life-Changing Magic of Tidying Up*. All around us, more and more ways of "going less" are popping up.

Before minimalism was a fad, I had already gotten rid of shoes that prevented the full movement of the thirty-three joints in each foot—shoes with heels of various heights, stiff soles, and not enough space for my toes to spread—and replaced them with footwear made of less material. I also spent less time in shoes overall. I made these changes for stronger feet and improved function of my entire body, but the way I did it—by putting more foot movement into the time I was already spending on walking—made getting movement easier for me time-wise.

Once I'd experienced the very immediate and wide-ranging benefits of this kind of "improvement through downsizing," I realized I could do this—change things about my life to fit more movement into the same period of time—in arenas beyond my shoe closet. This way of choosing tasks to best meet your needs, what I call "stacking your life," requires you to take stock of your needs, how they're currently being met, and how you're spending your time. After taking a look at what needs I had regarding my home, I found that warmth and coziness and protection from the elements are essential for me, but that the items (most of my furniture) preventing my knees, hips, and ankles from articulating fully were working against me—especially given I also had "do things to improve the mobility of my knees, hips, and ankles" on my daily to-do list.

I got rid of the bulk of my furniture—the couches and chairs in the living room, the chairs in the dining room (we still have a dining table; it just sits very low to the ground), and our conventional beds (I swapped twenty-four inches of box spring and mattress for three inches of futon). I still have home décor; I just decided to eliminate many of the conveniently placed items that were preventing the full use of numerous parts of my body. Just as people clean out their cupboards of junk food when they're ready to eat in a more nutritious way, I cleaned out my house when I was ready to move in a more nutritious way.

"Going minimal" in terms of furniture was a simple way to restructure my habitat. But to be clear, "going minimal" isn't my objective. Quite the opposite: My goal is to go maximal.

Perspective is everything, and we are often led by what's visible. And so we call a reduction—in furniture or the stiffness of conventional footwear or the amount of spending we do each month—minimalism. There's less stuff, or we've spent less, so it must be minimalism. There's less manufacturing needed, less material, less energy. Minimalism.

But what if we framed and named this reduction for what it can yield—in many cases, more movement, more awareness, more nature, more time with family and friends, more time in nature with family and friends. What if we reframed minimalism of stuff to be maximalism of our natural structure—a robust body within a robust community within a less-taxed environment?

How liberating would it be for our minds, so wired for acquisition, to recognize the abundance to be found within an empty room? What if approaching daily tasks, like stacking wood or going to the post office, with fewer of the tools and gadgets that make them physically easier and faster, actually afforded us the movement we desire and require?

We've mistaken *getting more stuff* for *getting more out of life*. Once we can fully see how often our possessions present a physical barrier to getting the essentials we require, taking action to change our lifestyle only makes taking action with our body that much easier.

NUTRIENT DENSE

Our diets, my friends, are unstacked.

For the bulk of the human timeline, humans subsisted on wild food acquired through their own physical labor. Stacked. From generation to generation, wisdom about what to eat, when to harvest, and how to harvest was transmitted from successful humans to the next generation, and in this way the "proof" regarding which foods to eat was in the pudding. Not that plants and fish and reptiles and bugs and mammals are pudding (I've eaten bugs on purpose, and they're nothing like pudding), but if someone eating the diet they were passing down to you was alive to teach you what to eat—without modern supplementation and medicine—that diet had already been (mostly) proven to meet the biological needs of a human. Stacked.

As we moved away from eating things that had been culti-vated and distributed naturally for thousands of years, we began to significantly change what we were eating, in terms of how much we ate and of what and in what time of year, ending up at a point where our diet was no longer meeting all our physiological needs. We were unstacking our diet, but we didn't know that at first.

It took hundreds of years using the scientific method (to unstack the plants and animals themselves) to recognize that some diseases were symptoms of a nutritional deficit and exactly which of the compounds found within food could treat them.

Because illness was and often still is explained relative to nutri-ents, we've developed a sort of nutrient-centric perspective[7] regarding food. Many of us know much more about the unstacked parts, the minerals and vitamins as extracted from their natural context that don't occur naturally outside of food, than we do about the plants and animals they are naturally packaged within.

From these parts we're formulating new things to be eaten. On one hand, when compared part to part, these whole foods and formulated foods could seem similar to each other, sort of like walking over terrain and walking on a treadmill can seem similar. Of course, they're also very different, but in a nutrient-centric culture those differences don't stand out as much. Especially since we've implied, through the way we've investigated food to date, that the foodstuffs surrounding vitamins and minerals are superfluous. The differences between food produced in nature and human-manufactured foods and their effects on the body have not been investigated much; manufactured foods are being qualified as food simply because they contain parts taken out of raw materials from nature.

When nature's parts are manufactured into a food product, the small mass of vitamins and minerals we're eating the item for also contains additives. The additives we prefer make food taste better and last longer on the shelf, and often include more energy (calories). When we package the nutrients we need with all the flavors and calories we can, the density of nutrients can go down while the number of empty calories goes up. Wild food—food that's shooting up from the ground, swimming down a river, dangling from a tree, and running overground—offers an abundance of nutrients without any added calories (i.e., it is nutrient-dense); the nutrients we get from our manufactured food products come in a big caloric package, as well as colorfully printed plastic, alongside many other similar, tempting foods in a brightly lit grocery store.

If you're numbers-savvy, you might have already gathered where I'm headed with this. In order to get the number of vitamins and minerals we have always needed, we'rse consuming unnaturally high numbers of calories (and often packaging) around those nutrients. This is largely due to our reliance on packaged food, and also because we've engineered and bred many of our whole foods to be less like their wild counterparts, to taste more sweet and less bitter. And our palates might prefer we get vitamin C from fruit rather than kale.

When you couple this diet of foods poor in nutrient density with a huge dose of food-related sedentarism (we don't move to grow, harvest, process, or even chew most of what we eat), it's likely you'll find yourself whole-body malnourished. The math is simple: If you have to decrease your calories consumed to match your low levels of movement throughout the day, every day, and the foods you know to eat are low in nutrients given the calories they contain, then you'll wind up with fewer nutrients than you require. Or if you eat to gather your required nutrients, you'll be overfed in terms of calories.

From Harvard Health Publications, a division of Harvard Medical School:

> [M]any of us doubt whether we can get all the nutrients we need from food alone. For one thing, the "percent daily values" featured on food labels are based on a 2,000-calories-a-day diet. Many of us can't eat that much without gaining weight. What if your energy needs are closer to 1,500 calories a day? What if you're dieting? Can you eat enough to take in the recommended micronutrients without falling back on a multivitamin?[8]

(Dear Harvard website, if you can stack your thinking here, you'll see that if one changed one's focus solely from nutrients to the types of foods they were eating to get them and measured just how little they were moving and corrected for sedentarism, this issue would right itself. See "Stack Your Life" on page 134.)

Our nutrient-centricism means we've created a hierarchy of what's most important about food, and the nutrients we've extracted are at the top. This isn't surprising given that our relationship with nutrients is a medical one. We haven't used our new understanding that the foods we eat as a culture don't meet our needs to change how we go about feeding ourselves; we've just turned that knowledge toward creating a necessary medicine for the way we continue to live. And the plants and animals that provide the raw materials for whole and manufactured foods are, it should be noted, simply those we've found to be easiest to produce. The foods that we consider foundational to our diets might not be the best for our bodies as much as they are the easiest to mass produce. Maybe ease (or mass production, for that matter) isn't nature's way at all, and through just a bit more of our own personal legwork, we'd find, right beneath our feet, plants and animals that nourish us better than the limited options currently presented to us.

Though they have tremendous value, nutrients don't work in a vacuum. Each nutrient works differently when packaged with other nutrients and, as you can imagine, with other organisms in the ecosystems, like bugs and bacteria. These natural interactions are lost in most manufactured processes. Individually, we cannot survive on vitamins and minerals alone, and collectively we cannot survive on knowledge vitamins—the small bits of understanding we have about what we eat. We have an extensive list of all the nutrients we need and all the food that contains them, so our knowledge seems vast. But this long list of facts masks that we've yet to consider more complex models of food that would meet our needs without food-parts-as-medicine and reduce the way our food system strains the ecosystem. We don't yet see how or where we source our individual diets as a part of what makes (or breaks) the nourishment available to our species, collectively.

For hundreds of thousands of years, the wisdom of how to eat sufficiently in a sustainable way has been handed down from one generation to the next. Currently standing in for elders in our culture is science, which is, relatively speaking, an infant in all matters of nature, currently informed only about which aspects of a food a body requires physiologically and, separately, which foods *of the ones they've decided to test* (again, we're most knowledgeable about the foods that we've found easiest to produce) contain these nutrients.

The information we get regarding our diet is not food wisdom. It's not "Here are the plants in your area to eat now, and here is the part that you can eat and the part you can't, and let me show you how to harvest this plant specifically, and here are some other plants you can harvest now and here's how to process them so they're not rancid later when there is no food; and don't eat that, as it's poisonous unless you feel ill here, in which case it's okay; and harvest this fish, but not that one because this first one has more fat, which indicates that it's not spawning,[9] so win-win, more energy for us and less detrimental to the fish population." Our diet information is just a limited collection of facts about the foods currently utilized in our culture.

We're able to get our food without much work, from anywhere in the world, at any time of year. And so instead of being from a local source (that we could move our bodies to gather ourselves), our nutrients come from far and wide in a way that often reduces the future availability of the nutrients. Our diet has quickly become inefficient.

Compared to eating processed foods with little nourishment and taking a multivitamin, eating a whole-food diet is one way to better stack your life. To stack further, to make your diet serve not only your needs better but also the needs of the planet, you could recognize that despite their wholeness, your foods might be unstacked in the sense that they're coming from far away, and their costs, in terms of the movement of others and taxes to the environment, are quite high, and that way of eating is ultimately working against you or your family in a broader sense. So eating seasonally or locally is another way to stack. Learning to incorporate the wild foods in your local area, the foods no one is eating any longer but that once upon a time, everyone in that area ate, is to stack it further still.

All this, perhaps unsurprisingly to you by now, relates back to movement. All the studies you read on "sitting is the new smoking" and "does stretching work?" and "which corrective exercises are the best for knee osteoarthritis?" are part of the same approach scientists have used when studying food—they're trying to figure out which movement nutrients eradicate which expressions of poor movement nutrition. We're working backwards, studying people in space, sedentary populations, sedentary populations that exercise, and active people who have certain weaknesses within otherwise fit bodies, to figure out which types of movement nourish which tissues. In other words, we're doing the same thing to movement that we've done to food—unstacking it.

It's clear our bodies need to move, but the idea that we *require* movement—that certain diseases erupt in a lack of either whole-body movement or the movement of a part within an area—is new. For the last fifty years, we've been working backwards to see which movements we humans actually need so we can then have our master list of necessary isolated movements to go with our vitamins and minerals. Like we divide diet into carbohydrates, fats, and proteins, we've divided movement into cardio, strength, and flexibility. Of course there are foods that contain protein, carbs, and fats, and there are also ways of moving that challenge our heart, muscles, and connective tissue all at once. But just as we've grown up not knowing what's edible around us and thus shop to import a narrow range of foods grown elsewhere, we don't know what movements are natural to our body. So we multitask daily at the gym—plucking vitamin Kegel and vitamin Calf Stretch, vitamin Ab Workout, vitamin Upper-Body Day (which we are careful to balance with vitamin Lower-Body Day) off our master list, and using them like supplements. Or we pick a single category of movement nutrient, like cardio, and consume that category of movement exclusively. This way of moving is not only poor in terms of nutrition, it's also inefficient.

Nutrient-dense food and nutrient-dense movement are packaged elegantly in nature. Or more accurately, there is no fluff when it comes to nature. The foods and the movements created, together, by nature are the essentials. These wild parts *are* the nutrients in a much larger picture, on a much grander scale.

7. Schuldt, J.P., and A.R. Pearson. 2015. "Nutrient-Centrism and Perceived Risk of Chronic Disease." *Journal of Health Psychology* 20(6): 899–906. doi: 10.1177/1359105315573446.

8. Harvard Health Publications. 2009. "Getting Your Vitamins and Minerals Through Diet." *Harvard Medical School*, July. <health.harvard.edu/womens-health/getting-your-vitamins-and-minerals-through-diet>

9. Rouja, Philippe M., Éric Dewailly, Carole Blanchet, and the Bardi Community. 2003. "Fat, Fishing Patterns, and Health Among the Bardi People of North Western Australia." *Lipids* 38: 399. doi:10.1007/s11745-003-1075-z.

GEESE, OR MOVEMENT ECOLOGY

When I consider the facts I have about human movement, I'll often consider other groups of animals in nature to get a broader picture before I jump in.

For example, many birds fly. Many also soar, glide, walk, perch, and float or swim, but for now let's just say I'm most interested in how they fly. If I wanted to quantify how a goose flies in order to understand and explain the natural movement of this bird, I would follow practices used for the study of human movement and begin with something easy, like examining how the goose uses its wings. I would count how often it beats its wings and which angles each wing moves through while it flies past my lab, and figure out which muscles are being used for goose flight. I could present this model in research titled "How a Goose Flies."

But of course flying is not a spontaneous arrival in the air. The takeoff and landing phases that bookend time in the air are part of the flying phenomenon. There is no flying without the takeoff and landing; the takeoff part and the landing part of flying don't operate similarly to each other or to the way the goose holds steady at altitude. Including these phases in my (fake) research brings me a step closer to accurately modeling and thus understanding the phenomenon of goose flight.

If I widened my observation of flying geese beyond my local goose pond, I would notice that the mechanics of how a goose flies—which muscles it uses to lift its legs or move one or both wings and in which way and how much—varies depending on temperature or the goose's height above the earth or the winds created by mountain ranges. Thus the season and geography impact the location and frequency of the muscle use of a goose, including how and how often it uses its wings while traveling over different landscapes and in different temperatures (soaring at high altitudes is one way to keep cool). I could add these observations to my compilation of research, still titled "How a Goose Flies."

If I wanted to be even more accurate—and why wouldn't I?—I would, at some point, need to expand my research to include the observation that birds most often fly in groups, and in particular in formations within a group. Each bird takes time in a lead position, using its body in a particular way to fly harder (this goose *moves the wind*) while the others use their bodies in a particular way to capitalize on the work being done in the front (these geese sort of *ride the wind*). The lead then falls back to rest while another assumes the work to benefit the group. The way a goose flies depends on, among the other factors I've listed above, its position within a group, which changes over short periods of time. I could call my expanded research—you guessed it—"How a Goose Flies."

These are all examples of mechanical ways to approach the study of goose flight. But what about the impetus of goose flight—what makes it go in the first place? Is it hunger? Can geese sense their food supply? Are they interacting with it somehow? What about temperature and other signals given by the season? Geese are often taught to fly by their parents, so how do parents with abundant food expose their offspring to flying (or not)? What about magnetoreceptors and cryptochromes in the eyes and brains of migratory birds?[10] Now we have to add parts that previously might have been thought of as "non-movement-related" anatomy. The fact of the matter is, despite what is pulled out for a particular investigation and presented in an individual research paper, these understandings of a part work, much like a goose, when integrated into a flock of information. An entire bird, the entire flock, and the entire planet is part of "How a Goose Flies."

When I think of all the details that need to be added into information regarding human movement, I get excited. Science is the process through which we can better understand natural phenomena. However, when we forget just how many details there are in a phenomenon, it's easy to over-apply facts gathered from early studies to all movement of all humans everywhere rather than remembering the scenario to which those details apply.

When I was an undergraduate, I had a textbook that stated there were three kinds of human movement: dance, athletics, and fitness. It didn't occur to me that there were any other types of movement; and when I did start considering walking from point A to point B to be movement (obviously!) it didn't occur to me that this type of movement was beneficial in any way. I had been conditioned by the academics in charge of the knowledge comprising the science of kinesiology (the study of human movement) to think (and move) in terms of exercise because dance, athletics, and fitness were all they had been researching.

Of course, the textbook I read was wrong; there are many types of movement that aren't dance, athletics, or fitness. Once I realized the bias I had been taught, I started thinking of movement in terms of geometry (the frequency and burdens created by all the various shapes the body could assume) and leaving the mode (the type of exercise) out of it.

On a recent tour of the Museum of Flight near Seattle, Washington, I read this on a placard:

Birds fly in V formation to conserve energy. Could aircraft do the same? The leading bird in the V creates an upward current of air behind it. The next bird rides this updraft for free lift. The birds take turns being the leader. The U.S. Air Force and Boeing have tested whether aircraft could save fuel by flying in a V formation, like birds. Tests of C-17 cargo airplanes showed that formation flight could cut fuel consumption 10–20 percent.

My biomechanics-brain was instantly intrigued. I've long been interested in the idea that a group of humans moving together could affect the muscle usage of each individual. Cyclists likely know this and use this phenomenon regularly, but what about humans moving naturally? Does moving through nature as a group change how you do it, and does moving this way improve the biological success of the human as a species? When moving through natural terrain (full of grass, sticks, lumps, and bumps), the person in the lead is often reducing your workload by performing the work necessary to move or temporarily trample obstacles, and everyone else gets a break. Once, a woman asked me the best way to arm-carry her baby (vs. using a baby-carrying device) while walking, because the way she was doing it hurt her back. After showing her how to adjust her rib and pelvic alignment to better utilize and strengthen her muscles, I pointed out that additional alignment points would include the ribs, pelvis, and arms of another person—to share some of the work that would ultimately strengthen the group.

The sign I'd want to put up in my museum of human movement, if I had one, would probably read:

Birds fly in V formation to conserve energy. Could humans do the same? The leading bird in the V creates an upward current of air behind it. The next bird rides this updraft for free lift. Similarly, I can spend a lot more time moving outside if someone will carry my baby for me for a while so I can expend less energy while moving, and as my kids grow older, I can reciprocate by carrying another's child, thus allowing all of us—of all ages and strengths—to get more movement throughout the day.

When it comes to nature, most of us understand the idea that animals use movement—specific types of it—to survive. We're less used to considering ourselves as animals being affected by the same natural laws governing every other species. While we have movement scientists researching movement, biologists and ecologists and conservationists could be doing for humans what many seem intent on doing for the rest of the natural world: detailing natural movement for better understanding of a species (or at least how to keep them from extinction due to the environment we've been creating).

It has only been recently, relatively speaking, that humans have stopped moving in packs through nature (though they're endangered, there are still a few groups moving this way today, and there were slightly more groups doing it a mere century ago). Despite the science that demonstrates humans move in a group in nature, most scientists, movement professionals, and movers alike have yet to expand their way of thinking about movement beyond the first iteration of my fake research above, so that "How a Human Moves" is currently limited to a few parts of the human body, a few scenarios of movement, and thus only a few parts of the entire phenomenon that is a moving human. Even less helpful in the process of gathering facts necessary to understand the natural phenomenon of human movement is that most current human movement studies are the equivalent of studying captive or non-migratory geese without explicitly noting that the particular specimens being observed are outliers in terms of natural behavior.

If science is indeed the pursuit of knowledge of nature, it is time to begin thinking about movement from an ecological perspective. It's time to include humans moving in different societies when we detail human movement; time to consider the impact of a habitat on movement and the impact of movement on a habitat; and likewise the relationship between the needs of a society and the needs of a human body. This is movement ecology.

Assisted by the comparison of natural goose behavior to nonnatural goose behaviors—like how goose movements are being changed through human interaction and a loss of habitat—ecologists are learning what is unsustainable for the geese. The next step is to broaden our understanding of animals to include humans, and recognize that what is unsustainable for the goose is also unsustainable for the gander. I mean, human.

---

10. Public Library of Science. 2007. "Do Migratory Birds 'See' the Magnetic Field?" ScienceDaily, October 1. <sciencedaily.com/releases/2007/09/070926140836. htm>

NATURAL MOVEMENT IS EFFICIENT

There are many things we use movement for. We use it to strengthen our bodies, to offset disease, to look good, to feel relaxed, to feel tense, to get from A to B, to complete the actions that comprise our daily living, to be functional in the ways we need to be functional, to experience the world in the ways that we choose. But your physiology uses the movements you do for its own purpose: to operate.

Once upon a time, movement was natural and served multiple purposes. The first was to accomplish all tasks necessary to living in the wilderness—walking long distances over natural terrain, climbing, digging, clearing, scrambling, squatting, carrying, chopping, pulling, and sprinting, to name just a few. The movements done to accomplish these tasks not only reaped the reward of the task (climbing to pick fruit gave you fruit), but also another purpose of movement—adaptation, i.e., the development of the structure to do these tasks again and again, successfully (climbing to pick fruit made you better at climbing to pick fruit, thus increasing your ability to get more fruit). Beyond the benefits of accomplishing tasks and developing the structure to continue to do them, moving your whole body in this natural way was serving yet another purpose. Whole-body movement was moving the smaller parts of your body—the cells that make up the body (climbing to pick fruit uses certain body parts and moves the cells in those areas).

The small movements of each cell that happen when you move are themselves part of the physiological process that regenerates and maintains those moving parts. Movement, just like the cell wall, the mitochondria, the cytoskeleton, and the nucleus, *is a part of every working cell.* Cells don't work without movement, and you aren't fully operational without all of your cells working well. The movement of a part today is what affords it the ability to move tomorrow, but make sure you read the fine print on this uber-efficient deal: many of the benefits of movement are local to the working part.[11]

We can talk about the total movement we do each day, but first we need deeper clarification regarding movement. It's not only that you need to move more often than you do right now; you also need to move *more of you* more often than you do right now.

We've got a nice foundation of understanding when it comes to the idea that a flourishing body is made up of mostly strong parts rather than a lot of strength in just a few. Cross-training—mixing up your movements to use more body parts—for better performance and less injury has been recommended for some time now. Physical therapy is an entire profession dedicated to assessing which parts of you are working too little or too much and providing exercises and geometries of movement (also known as "form") to isolate unworking (or excessively working) parts to reduce injury, pain, and the risk of it happening again. The problem is, perhaps without realizing it, we've been using movement in the same way we've used dietary supplements.

The process of investigating movement is very similar to the process we're currently using with food and nutrients. There's a movement diet, so to speak, and it's not nourishing us fully; there are diseases and ailments erupting in groups of humans who move certain ways (or don't at all). We're trying to figure out how to spot-treat each person with different movement vitamins while missing a larger issue altogether: Our culturally approved ways of moving aren't meeting our needs.

Just like we've been told we need protein, fat, and carbs, we know we need cardio, strength, and flexibility. We're told we need to train our upper and lower body and core muscles for the best outcome. As with food, we're missing wisdom when it comes to movement. The bulk of the exercises we're told to do are human-made. They contain elements of nature—an elbow bend, an extended hip, an arched back—but they're blended with other motions, specially manufactured equipment, a special building, required footwear, and the right outfit. Our exercises are just like processed food. They're not necessarily the most nutritious; they're just the easiest for us to produce within our sedentary lifestyle. They're all that we know to eat because we come from a sedentary culture where there's hardly anyone left to hand down the practice of movement.

Just as all the organic, nutrient-dense materials we needed to make food were once at our fingertips, so were all the organic, nutrient-dense movements that acquired that food. And those were a lot of movements. Not three or ten or even fifty whole-body movements, but more movement and movements than you can probably imagine.

We're finding it difficult to be nourished by exercise as we do it today, because not only is it infrequent (you know you need to move more, yes?) but also, although the whole body can benefit to a point when only some parts are working, the exercises we're choosing work *very* few of our parts. Practically speaking, the answer we're looking for isn't only to the question "How can I find the time to move more?" but also to "How can I find the time to move *all of my parts* more?"

You can move each part one at a time, or a few of them at a time, which is what most of us do when we exercise, but the degree of health (and future movement) generated by this approach is limited by time. There's simply no time to move all your trillions of parts at a natural frequency when your way of moving uses a few parts at a time a small percentage of each day.

But there's something else to consider, too. (Isn't there always?)

Before I began thinking like an ecologist, I was a proponent of natural movements simply because they're so numerous and varied in form. Natural-movements-for-exercise use many more parts of the body than isolated exercises do—making them a more efficient way of reaching the greatest number of parts. Yes, these movements were sort of archaic in the modern world, but they were of great design—definitely superior to any exercise I could craft on the gym floor. Archaic, but efficient.

What I've come to realize is that natural movements are not archaic at all. They are still the motions required to get life's necessities. We have not eliminated the need for these human movements; we've simply given them to someone else to do. Natural movements are only perceived as archaic by the group of people who have outsourced them.

So here we are. We need to move more, we need to move more of us. We need to fit more movement into our lives and, for the sake of ourselves and other humans, we need to reclaim some of the necessary movements we've outsourced. Which brings me back to natural movement. Natural movements are not just how cave people moved; they're the movements that bring about a structure able to walk short and long distances; find, gather, and process our own food; carry the burden of our own stuff. Natural movements are parts of a functioning ecosystem that includes humans.

Though we've been able to outsource the movements necessary to reap the rewards of movement, we haven't been able to outsource our need for the movement of each of our parts. This is why a daily bout of exercise of some parts does not nourish us fully.

Exercise is unstacked movement. Not only are we trying to make our bodies better part by part, but also we're using movement to improve only one part of our lives—our physical structure and health.

If we think about things ecologically, we need a way to exercise that best prepares our body to perform more of our own necessary tasks. We need a way of moving that, while improving our ability to execute functional tasks—to be able to walk longer distances safely and pain-free, to carry our own things and children, to squat, bend, and dig in our yards for a portion of our food—also allows us to take each of our cells to the repair shop to get a tune-up. We need a stacked way of moving.

You know what I'm going to say next, don't you?

Natural movement is long-established and ultra-efficient in these matters. Refined over millennia, natural movement is the natural phenomenon that facilitates both our personal movement and our non-movement needs, naturally.

---

11. Lindholm, M. E., F. Marabita, D. Gomez-Cabrero, et al. 2014. "An Integrative Analysis Reveals Coordinated Reprogramming of the Epigenome and the Transcriptome in Human Skeletal Muscle After Training." *Epigenetics* 9(12): 1557–1569.

NATURAL MOVEMENT IS JOYFUL

Becoming as competent at moving through nature as is possible for you is not only about achieving the movements or reaping the physiological and tangible rewards of the movements. There are also experiences that only natural movements in nature can afford. For example, squatting can do more than open your hips; the ability to squat opens up how you see the world. A squat puts a different part of the world in front of your face and reveals more of it—stuff you can't see and interact with unless you get down to the ground and look closely.

On a recent trip to New Mexico a squat facilitated the chance to inspect tiny succulents, plants only visible once I was down there, with my kids, poking through the rocks on the desert floor. We miss so many little things when we always take in the world from the same height, from the same perspective.

Likewise, prioritizing the work to develop a more stable gait and quick reflexes as you move over ground with its natural lumps and bumps and slipperiness and shape doesn't just result in strong feet and ankles and good balance. Strong parts gift us the ability to move with enough confidence to not constantly watch the ground ahead of us. We can look up and around at the world that surrounds us.

And it's not only the big stuff like moving hips and knees and shoulders and spines this former lover of "big exercises" has found delightful. The smaller motions of weaving, molding pottery, crushing spices, cracking nuts, and picking berries are big in the satiation they offer the non-physical part of me that created something new—a necessity that I, until then, had only experienced as something I bought ready-made. On my personal journey of training my body and lifestyle towards more natural movement, it's not the thirty-seven-mile walkabout I did one day that has brought me the most joy, but the day I learned how to create cordage by braiding the fibers of grass and nettle. String and rope, it turns out, are key to survival in nature (and also free jewelry)!

Grand motions and small gestures, huge physical feats and tiny triumphs can all offer experiences of accomplishment, self-efficacy, confidence, and glee. The accumulation of natural movements used for producing some necessity is a tapestry of satisfaction being woven in our minds just as much as in our cells.

MOVEMENT IS COUNTER-CULTURE

Out of all the nutrients we require, dietary, movement, and other, perhaps none is as essential to the sustainability of our bodies and of all humanity as the awareness vitamin. Giving thoughtful consideration to ideas and paying attention to the words used to express them when you're reading and listening are crucial.

I once read a research paper[12] discussing microbiologist René Dubos's writings (his books are fabulous and I highly recommend them) on the state of modern humans and the implications of a world filled with rapidly developing technologies.

> Dubos argued that because humans are very adaptable, the relationship between an evolutionary mismatch and erosion of health would be stealth-like; there would be only minimal awareness of the association, especially early on in the era of high technology and urbanization. In other words, it would be difficult for the general population and even health-care providers to make connections between current ill health and exceeding adaptive limits in the years or decades prior. Moreover, since humans are also attracted to gadgets and, as Dubos argued, *"seem to accept willingly, and indeed to enjoy"* many of the biological stresses of mega-city life, it would be even more difficult to appreciate ancestral needs that might be *missed* in the modern environment.
>
> According to Dubos, humans, as a species, would make the necessary adaptations for *survival* in the technological and increasingly urbanized environment. However, survival could not be equated to optimal health or quality of life, and such adaptations

may not be without cost to the individual and ultimately to society. The detrimental health effects
of the slow and insidious presence of physical and
psychological toxins, disturbed circadian rhythms,
artificial foodstuffs (all acting in concert with the
absence of nature interaction), would bypass iden-
tification by most individuals—rather, according to
Dubos, they would only be apparent in the overall
health statistics of the larger nature-disconnected
population over time.

I've thought about these paragraphs a lot. At first, I couldn't figure out how a science-based society with a track record of mind-boggling technologies developed out of their great obser- vational skills could be simultaneously oblivious to the impact of those technologies. But then I started paying closer attention.

In 2015, a study[13] came out about grip strength and how a lack of it correlated to all-cause mortality, cardiovascular mortality, non-cardiovascular mortality, myocardial infarction, stroke, and, in high-income countries, a risk of cancer. The end application of this information was that a clinician could better predict cardiovascular and all-cause mortality by grip strength than by blood pressure. I wouldn't be surprised if there were also a boost in hand-strength- ener sales, given the media's spin—that hand strength is the ticket to longevity. (And, P.S., If you want to take a reading break and use your hands, if only to wring out this book a little bit, I'll wait.)

Why grip strength makes such a good predictor hasn't been investigated yet, but the working hypothesis is probably as you figured—that those with the strongest hands tend to move their entire bodies more. With apologies to anyone who ran out and bought the aforementioned hand strengtheners, it's unlikely that having *only* strong hands is protective. So parlay that enthusiasm into whole-body activities that use your hands, and boom! You'll be in it to win it. Win at strengthening your hands and your other parts too, that is.

A study that came out the following year showed that in 2016, American men younger than thirty and women ages twenty to twenty-four have significantly weaker hand grip strength than their counterparts twenty years before. Men's strength losses ran in the 14–16-pound (6–7 kg) range (grip strength in 1985 was over 100 pounds, or 45 kg) and women's losses averaged around 10 pounds (4.5 kg), from 70 pounds (31.7 kg) in 1985 to 60 pounds (27.2 kg) in 2016. In terms of percentages, these losses translate to a 10 percent decrease in grip strength in men and a 14 percent decrease in women.

As far as biological norms go, this is a tremendous loss in function, and when I read it I saw it immediately as important data regarding the impact of lifestyle and habitat on biological performance. Which is why I was surprised to see the application of this understanding of nature to be that *the norms of strength clearly need to be lowered.* According to NPR, who reported the findings in a piece titled "Millennials May be Losing Their Grip":[14]

> Like fashion trends, co-author Fain says healthcare norms should be updated roughly every 10 years. That makes handgrip measurement well overdue for reassessment.
>
> In other words, the 1985 norms may belong in a drawer—replaced but not forgotten—along with leg warmers, Swatches and scrunchies.

And there it is—the idea, from the researchers themselves, that the norms of biological performance should be adjusted to match how humans of a particular lifestyle behave. Fortunately, science isn't how a society chooses to interpret the data collected; it is simply all the data.

Michael Pollan wrote a fascinating book called *The Omnivore's Dilemma*, wherein he documents the cost, in terms of "fossil fuel calories," of four different meals: fast food from McDonald's, an entire "big organic" meal from Whole Foods, a meal cooked with ingredients from a small farm, and a meal including many ingredients he hunted and foraged himself.

At the end of the book, he dismisses the practicality of both the fast-food meal and the foraged meal: "Let us stipulate that both of these meals are equally unreal and equally unsustainable. Which is perhaps why we should do what a responsible social scientist would do under the circumstances: discard them both as anomalies and outliers—outliers of a real life."

While I believe that Pollan is simply saying it would be impractical for most people to head out and hunt and gather their meals (likely due to a lack of skill, knowledge, and wild spaces at this point), the idea that it's irresponsible for science to even *present* this way of eating as an option for humans to consider working towards, via a lot of collective work and transition time, of course, is itself, well, irresponsible.

It's like continuing to prescribe stiff, supportive footwear for foot health rather than strengthening the feet themselves simply because we've cultivated weak feet and covered the earth with human-made surfaces and debris. It's like saying that continuing to recommend breastfeeding to women who live in a society that requires they go out and make money to buy necessities is irresponsible. These examples suggest that what *is* responsible is to perpetuate the environment that leads to decreasing grip strength, diseased feet, great distancing from our food, and imparting unstacked nutrition to our offspring.

Like a culture in a petri dish, cultures (and corporations, for that matter) are occupied with perpetuating themselves and require every cell on board for that to happen. It requires an indoctrination system that brings us to the point where we feel social scientists need to disregard biological sciences and make things like food and movement social issues, not physiological ones. It requires that we view change as something that happens on a large scale first (brought about by government institutions and policies) rather than what change actually is: the transition, over time, of many people making small changes in habit. It requires a widely held perception that it's *irresponsible* to suggest the essentialness of any behavior that falls outside the norms of the culture in which we currently operate. Heck, it's not even about social science at this point. Pollan, in his own poetic description of what was "at least for [him], the perfect meal," names the meal itself as "a wordless way of saying grace." Pollan is tuned in to the vitality of eating the body of the world, but then says it's simply unreal (see my thoughts on what's real or not on pages 120–121), meaning what? That it's too hard? Is this about responsibility, or is it about sedentarism? (No offense, M.P.; you do great work and we're all in this together.)

Movement, this essential part of our health and survival, has become counter-culture, as have many of the other elements we need, leading to adaptations that are not in favor of us continuing as a society, or as a species—just as Dubos predicted. To carry on ignoring known mechanisms of nature because continuing to be a sedentary society is more *practical* is the truly irresponsible (and unsustainable) position.

12. Logan, A.C., M.A. Katzman, V. Balanza-Martinez. 2015. "Natural Environments, Ancestral Diets, and Microbial Ecology: Is There a Modern 'Paleo-Deficit Disorder'? Part I." *Journal of Physiological Anthropology* 34:1. <jphysiolanthropol.biomedcentral.com/articles/10.1186/s40101-015-0041-y>

13. Leong, D. P., K.K. Teo, S. Rangarajan et al. 2015. "Prognostic Value of Grip Strength: Findings from the Prospective Urban Rural Epidemiology (PURE) Study." *The Lancet* 386(9990): 266–273. <thelancet.com/journals/lancet/article/PIIS0140-6736(14)62000-6/abstract>

14. Jacewicz, N. 2016. "Millennials May Be Losing Their Grip." *Shots: Health News From NPR*, June 13. <npr.org/sections/health-shots/2016/06/13/481590997/millennials-may-be-losing-their-grip>

MOVEMENT IS NOT MEDICINE

Our family enjoys an occasional trip to the zoo, but sometimes we end up inadvertently learning more about human animals than about monkeys and elephants. On one memorable visit to the Santa Barbara Zoo I read a sign titled "Pedicures for Pachyderms" posted outside an elephant exhibit:

> Our elephants receive foot care as part of their daily routine. Healthy and well-maintained feet are essential to the overall well-being and longevity of elephants. Just like you would trim your dog's or cat's nails, we do the same with [our elephants]. Every day the elephants soak their feet and then the keepers hose them down, scrub them, moisturize them, and apply disinfectant. About once a week the keepers do a more extensive session where they file and trim the elephants' nails and pads as well.

I found this sign to be a good lesson in perspective and how easy it is to leave off "because caged elephants are not moving an appropriate amount or over natural terrain, and foot disease was a leading cause of death in captive elephants before they started giving them walks and pedicures"[15] when delivering information on these particular elephants.

I used to say "movement is medicine." I even wrote an essay titled this once. But the more understanding I have, the less I agree with the phrase. Now, from the get-go I'll say that I myself was trained in a therapy-centric science and that I personally teach and will continue to teach corrective exercise and what could be considered movement therapy. But my therapy perspective exists in a larger, non-therapy-centric model, that is, a model of health that doesn't frame the therapy—a treatment that can be more costly and "unstacked" than the organic occurrences in nature it is derived from—as "necessary for human health."

We're in a pickle, because we're in desperate need of solutions to a problem that we have, so far, been unwilling or unable to identify; or perhaps we're entirely aware of it and just leave it off the signs we're posting about humans. We're animals who require nature who are living out of nature, and we are looking for a way to flourish in captivity. However, there is a difference between what a human requires and what it takes to keep from dying in captivity. Not that we don't benefit from the latter, but confusing them won't help us understand the part of nature that is human.

The needs of a society dictate the pursuit of science, and right now we are most interested in therapy models necessary for our type of society. This need often replaces a pursuit for human-physiology models describing necessary inputs for movement, diet, sunlight, human-to-human interactions, etc. We're overwhelmed with the need for the therapies and so, without a working knowl-edge of natural human behavior, we opt for supplements in lieu of a nutrient-rich diet and abundant outdoor time, exercises in lieu of a movement-rich life, and professional touch therapies in lieu of family or tribal touch. This isn't a criticism of therapy models; I find value in bodywork sessions, I still teach corrective exercise, and I think people can beneficially use the assistance of the amazing therapies we have developed. But it's essential to consider that the tendency of a sedentary culture might be to parlay scientific facts into amazing therapeutic practices that allow it to stay sedentary, rather than to assemble that same data in a way that clearly demonstrates the tremendous amounts of therapy it takes for us to function.

Therapies help us function in our cultural context, and I'm not suggesting the therapies themselves need to change. But we've begun to perceive that our pelvic floor problems stem from not doing our Kegel exercises, rather than from our lifetime of inadequate movement; and that our vitamin D deficiency has arisen from our not taking enough vitamin D tablets, rather than from a lifestyle that keeps us most frequently indoors[16] or eating a diet that changes the effect of the sun on our bodies.[17] We're mistaking the therapy for the need.

The transition in a patient or therapy-offering practitioner's mindset could be as simple as "this therapy is replacing natural behavior X, so supplement with this for now, and here are some strategies for getting more behavior X in your life and therefore less therapy."

In my own career as an instructor of exercise, while I have always taught useful exercises that many have found helped various parts of their bodies to function better, I found over and over again that once helped, they wanted even more exercises. This was great, because they were finally able to move, and wanted to move even more. But soon everyone had a list of a hundred exercises that they couldn't fit into each day and had to constantly pick the health of one body part over another. Finally, I had to say to myself, enough with presenting only correctives, it's time to stack these parts back into their natural context. I reframed my presentation as I've noted before: These correctives are aspects of much larger, much easier-to-integrate-into-your-life movements that nourish a whole lot more of you when you do many of them at once.

The number of movement supplements (i.e., corrective exercises) it takes to make a whole body, a whole family, and a whole lifetime of strength is too many when broken down into smaller parts. An efficient use of dietary supplements is to use them to decrease your symptoms so that you can transition into someone who knows what foods to eat, where to get them, and how to prepare them. Using that model, I decided it would be more efficient, for me and for those wanting to know "all the exercises" and "all the things improved by movement," to teach exercises that would help people function well enough to move their bodies more often, and more often in nature, where, just like wild food, the nutrient density is higher—because of the terrains, textures, natural light, nature sounds, and randomness of it all. Nature is the ultimate instructor of whole-body movement.

Inadvertently, our culture is reinforcing the idea that humans don't have what it takes to be healthy, but that they can be saved through therapy. Even the idea that nature is therapy stems from the idea that nature isn't our natural state, which it is.

Movement isn't medicine. Pedicures are medicine. Weekly pedicures necessary to prevent death are a sign that needs heeding. When things don't move well, other people and tools are needed to do what would otherwise happen naturally. Medicine is what you need when a rare issue arises in your life, not what you need to compensate for your lifestyle. Movement and food (and community and a community of bacteria and likely a host of other things) are *essentials*. Essentials are not medicine, they are not spot treatments; they are regularly required inputs.

I get it when people say movement is medicine. They mean, as I did, that we can, in many cases, use exercises to avoid medicine. But this only goes for the movements we understand. There are many other issues arising from a lack of movement that we wouldn't know how to remedy with a corrective exercise, because not a single corrective exercise, or even twenty of them together, could begin to address the complexity. It's time to post the sign in its entirety. We're sick, and so are many other aspects of nature, because we don't move. Movement is not medicine. Movement is essential.

15. Cohn, Jeffrey P. 2006. "Do Elephants Belong in Zoos?" *BioScience* 56(9): 714–717.

16. Godar, Dianne E., Robert J. Landry, and Anne D. Lucas. "Increased UVA Exposures and Decreased Cutaneous Vitamin D_3 Levels May Be Responsible for the Increasing Incidence of Melanoma." *Medical Hypotheses* 72(4): 434–443.

17. Liu, Guangming, Douglas M. Bibus, Ann M. Bode, Wei-Ya Ma, Ralph T. Holman, and Zigang Dong. 2001. "Omega 3 but Not Omega 6 Fatty Acids Inhibit AP-1 Activity and Cell Transformation in JB6 Cells." *PNAS* 98(13): 7510–7515.

VITAMIN COMMUNITY

One of the coolest things about skeletal anatomy is that once you know which shape each bone is, you can apply the knowledge to most of the vertebrates in the animal kingdom. Horse, whale, bird, dinosaur, human—a pelvis is pelvis-shaped, ribs are easily identified, and yep, that's a femur. Knowledge of the skeleton is easily transferred from animal to animal, which saves time when it comes to figuring things out about each individual animal. Where the lungs are isn't such a mystery. "Where does the baby come out?" doesn't need to be deduced every time.

Though not as tangible as the hardened minerals that comprise skeletal bone, there is a framework of nutrients or nutrient-esque essentials (all of the inputs that support us physically) that could be generalized as necessary to a wide variety of animals. Not that all animals require the same inputs (nor skeletons, for that matter). Bats have different dietary needs from whales, and some animals live in groups while others spend their adult lives in isolation. Still, the shape of a general nutrient framework—the well-researched facts demonstrating that there are essential habitats, diets, and social structures necessary to each animal—is sufficient to save us time when it comes to figuring out all that human animals require.

Nutrients are something our bodies need that our bodies either cannot manufacture at all or cannot manufacture in sufficient quantities. They cause our physiology to be altered when they are introduced to our bodies. When nutrients are missing or insufficient in a human body, the result is a disease or malfunction; thus, nutrients can only be identified once we understand that the experience we are having is a symptom arising from a lack of a necessity. This is a super-important point (Is it weird to write "super-important" in your own book? Probably, but I really want you to hear what I'm saying.): Nutrients are identified through hindsight, and this means we must pay close attention and document changes in groups of humans living in particular ways.

So, we have a current list of human nutrient needs. On the most general level, we say that humans need food and water and shelter, but clearly this is oversimplified. We don't need just food but nutrient-dense food. Our need for shelter is really how we meet our needs for warmth (or a stable temperature) and protection, and thus adequate rest. We also need to move (and to be moved), and what about sleep? Vitamin sleep is huge and I, for one, am sorely in need—clearly, since I've mentioned it twice in the last three sentences. Humans need gravity (our space studies show), and a flourishing microbiome, and natural light. And if we use our framework of animal needs and our understanding of how humans have succeeded historically, we find that humans need close contact with other humans.

Until very recently, the social structure of human animals has been organized by the same efficiency principles that organize everything in nature.[18] We lived in small groups (and perhaps groups within groups), where necessary work was shared. It wasn't in the way we share society's work today—unlike the honeybees, in mainstream Western culture right now we each struggle daily to execute all tasks necessary for a collective to survive. Each person is responsible for getting their own groceries, making their own meals, cleaning their own house, minding their own kids. Instead, our natural social structure used to be (and still is, in a few very discrete places) more like that of the trees. In nature the structure of society is stacked so that individuals work together, in a cooperative fashion, to regularly use their personal strengths to provide something to the group as well as shunt nutrients—especially in the form of food and childcare[19]—as the need arises.

Our historical use of community is hypothesized to be all about food and kids. Human animals have a long juvenile period. It takes a long time to learn how to eat from the wild. The adult humans in existing hunter-gatherer communities we can research aren't ever providing just childcare; children are always, even in their play, being exposed to skills that will parlay into food acquisition. *Moving* with adults who are gathering and processing food is also education for children on gathering and processing food, and it's healthcare for all. But it isn't only parents providing education and healthcare to their children. In a tribe, juvenile care (and thus education, movement, and touch) is provided by parents and also alloparents—grandparents, childless peers, other children. This arrangement is efficient in that it increases the child's chance for survival; gives purpose and contribution to elder tribal members and allows essential information to pass between generations; provides not-yet-parents the opportunity to be with children; and (I might be biased in my phrasing here, as a mother of two kids under the age of five) *saves* the primary parent from burnout. The parents of young children in a tribe, despite their status, are still required to go out and work for their food, much like we all have to in non-tribal societies. And did I mention the movement? At the heart of everything a tribe offers is all-day movement for everyone. Movement is nourishment and the amount of it goes up for all, especially in the case of young children, who require their initial movement be facilitated, when there are many hands to move and be moved.

A tribe is efficiently organized in that it utilizes local resources of people to directly meet the needs of all members of the group. A tribe is a stacked community.

For most of us today, our relationship with "others" is sort of like all of our relationships with other things from the natural world— separated into parts. Isolated and contained in separate locations are many of the elements a community offers: food, childcare, education, spiritual guidance, art, music, medicine, touch-therapy, eldercare, movement (in the form of exercise). We have all these parts because they are necessary elements of a human society, but they are certainly unstacked from the way nature originally organized human groups. I propose that the inefficiency of our modern situation might be hindering our ability to be fully nourished, either due to the time issue (i.e., there's no possible way to get everything we need when it's all separated), or because there's something more to the "whole" of an intact community, greater than the sum of its parts, that we don't yet understand.

Because of the reciprocity of nature, I suggest that as we outsourced movement to others beyond our local community (often to other countries), we decreased our need for immediate community. And as we stopped moving on behalf of ourselves and others, our sheer ability to move decreased, as did what we could contribute to a community. So now we're at the place where it's necessary for a sedentary society to get all the essential elements of community in separate parts. Which means that to continue to operate our current society this way is to continue to perpetuate a society that *requires* we stay sedentary.

If we're to transition back to a lifestyle that affords more movement—if we're going to stack our life for more movement—the community aspect must also work towards being stacked, *because that's how nature works.*

In addition to (and definitely related to) a lack of movement, there are many things almost all of us can relate to right now: feeling too busy, feeling too tired, feeling stretched in too many directions. Feeling as though there's something missing from our lives; spending money on things we don't need to try to fill the space left by the something that's missing. We're a large group of people all experiencing these troubling feelings. Depression, addiction, anxiety, loneliness, pain, and chronic illness are common in our culture, which is why I'm going to repeat my super-important point: *Nutrients are identified through hindsight, and this means we must pay close attention and document changes in groups of humans living in particular ways.*

To recognize human-to-human interaction as a nutrient, we must be able to identify the symptoms of a lack of it. Doesn't the list of shared experiences in our culture read like a list of symptoms? Another step in the investigative process would be to recognize when community, or elements found in a community, are being used successfully as a therapy for these ailments, a step that often precedes research on nutrients. For example, the discovery of vitamin C was made possible (two hundred years before any research) by those who figured out that oranges worked for treating scurvy symptoms before they knew why (emphasis mine):

The pioneering controlled clinical trial of the various therapies recommended for the disease of scurvy... was carried out in 1746 by James Lind on sailors at sea.... He took 12 sailors, all with a similar severity of the disease, divided them into pairs and, for 2 [weeks], gave each pair one of the many treatments that had been recommended for the condition.... The pair receiving lemons and oranges were almost recovered after only 6 d[ays], whereas those receiving either dilute sulfuric acid or vinegar had shown no improvement after 2 [weeks].

The importance of Lind's trial has often been described as showing that citrus fruit was a cure, or preventive, for scurvy. **This had, in fact, been known already for some 200 y[ears] but could not always be made use of.**[20]

I'm a proponent of "vitamin Community," but community might not even be the best word choice when it comes to investigating this human need, in the same way that saying we need "shelter" or "food" sells our actual needs a bit short. Our need for community could be delineated into a need to belong to something and to have something to contribute to. It could also be our need for touch, communication, support, and, you guessed it, more movement, making community a collection of nutrients.

As we recognize that community, or elements found in community, are successful in treatments of addiction[21] and depression,[22] and as we find touch therapy and movement to be effective in reducing the symptoms of chronic pain and other ailments, we must then ask: Do we need the therapy, or do humans simply require the inputs community offers in the same way we need nutrient-dense food?

If it's the latter, we can, with this understanding of nature, restructure our lives so that the symptoms of our malnutrition arising from a lack of certain community nutrients do not continue to manifest, and we can then decrease our need for ongoing therapy. We all had to learn the value of and skill set to eating a nutritious diet, and

DON'T JUST SIT THERE

I wouldn't want to discourage anyone from donating money or time to those in need or contributing to causes you feel passionate about, or any other non-movement forms of activism. This book itself is an act of movement activism that required large quantities of sedentary behavior on the part of yours truly. Clearly we are in a state where activism of all types is necessary, especially to gain attention for those beings and those issues currently ignored. Please, keep up or begin activism of all shapes and forms.

You can *also* be more active in your support for a cause through small acts throughout the day—support low-income populations by getting involved with community garden building or tending, glean local areas for produce to go to food banks, make your own foods or source ingredients to reduce the labor in areas that are known to use slavery which then gets converted into domestic and child abuse. Comb through the information available about the causes you feel passionate about. See how your personal actions can reduce the contribution to what you view as the problem. Note how your physical attention to these matters not only benefits the cause but also your body.

Activism is challenging for many in that it can be scary. Viewing the act of moving to better tend to your own needs as a way of taxing other people or the planet less is a way to make regular, daily activism practical and sustainable.

likewise, we can all transition to a way of organizing our time and community members in a way that nourishes us fully.

At the heart of our unstacked society is money standing in for movement. This allows us to shunt nutrients to one another in the form of dollars. At first glance this is helpful, because others desperately need more and many of us have it to give. However, shunting money instead of the actual needed nutrient leaves everyone in the society low in the currency of movement. Can you imagine if a tree in a forest shunted another tree in need of water a twenty-dollar bill and said, "Go get yourself some nutrients with this"? Money cannot stand in equally for the work performed by another, because there is energy lost in the exchange. The work for a tree to buy itself some water takes time and energy, and here's the rub—this scenario still requires another tree to gather and deliver it. So shunting money instead of your own labor, directly, to your community is really just super-inefficient from a biological standpoint. Neither you nor the person you are trying to assist is getting the full spectrum of the nutrients you both need.

In the end, society, like all other aspects of nature, is subject to the natural laws of the universe. You can't purchase a replacement for the "whole" of the community that you need. But you can do the work of finding, or creating, and then sustaining a community. You and everyone around you will be better off for it.

---

18. Hamilton, M. J., B. T. Milne, R. S. Walker, O. Burger, and J. H. Brown. 2007. "The Complex Structure of Hunter-Gatherer Social Networks." *Proceedings of the Royal Society B: Biological Sciences* 274(1622): 2195-2202. <ncbi.nlm.nih.gov/pubmed/17609186>

19. Dyble, M., J. Thompson, D. Smith et al. 2016. "Networks of Food Sharing Reveal the Functional Significance of Multilevel Sociality in Two Hunter-Gatherer Groups." *Current Biology* 26 (15): 2017–2021. <cell.com/current-biology/abstract/S0960-9822(16)30564-4>

20. Carpenter, Kenneth J. 2003. "A Short History of Nutritional Science: Part 1 (1785–1885)." *J. Nutr.* 133(3): 638–645.

21. Jason, Leonard A., Bradley D. Olson, Joseph R. Ferrari, and Anthony T. Lo Sasso. 2006. "Communal Housing Settings Enhance Substance Abuse Recovery." *American Journal of Public Health* 96(10): 1727-1729. doi: 10.2105/AJPH.2005.070839.

22. Wells, K. B., L. Jones, B. Chung et al. 2013. "Community-Partnered Cluster-Randomized Comparative Effectiveness Trial of Community Engagement and Planning or Resources for Services to Address Depression Disparities." *Journal of General Internal Medicine* 28(10): 1268–1278. <rd.springer.com/article/10.1007/s11606-013-2484-3>

Additional Sources

Hidaka, Brandon H. 2012. "Depression as a Disease of Modernity: Explanations for Increasing Prevalence." *Journal of Affective Disorders* 140(3): 205–214. doi.org/10.1016/j.jad.2011.12.036.

Hosseinbor, M., S. M. Y. Ardekani, S. Bakhshani, and S. Bakhshani. 2014. "Emotional and Social Loneliness in Individuals With and Without Substance Dependence Disorder." *International Journal of High Risk Behaviors and Addiction* 3(3): e22688.

Hrdy, Sarah Blaffer. 2011. *Mothers and Others: The Evolutionary Origins of Mutual Understanding.* Cambridge, MA: Belknap Press.

Junger, S. 2016. *Tribe: On Homecoming and Belonging.* New York and Boston: Hachette Book Group.

Lamb, Michael E., and Barry S. Hewlett. 2005. *Hunter-Gatherer Childhoods: Evolutionary, Developmental, and Cultural Perspectives.* New Jersey: Aldine Transaction.

Sarris, Jerome, A. O'Neil, C. E. Coulson, I. Schweitzer, M. Berk. 2014. "Lifestyle Medicine for Depression." *BMC Psychiatry* 14: 107. doi.org/10.1186/1471-244X-14-107

PERSONAL MISSION STATEMENT

My family, my body, and the great outdoors. These are the things I treasure and prioritize over everything else—but that wouldn't always have been clear had you witnessed the day-to-day activities I used to choose to do.

Decisions can be overwhelming, especially when we don't always have the luxury of time to make an extensive cost/benefit analysis. I once heard that every organization, whether a company, a non-profit, or a family, should have a mission statement. And that when it comes time to make a decision, you should evaluate the decision against the mission statement in order to keep your organization true to its purpose.

As a lover of alignment of the body and the mind, I was instantly smitten with the idea. An external way to check if my behavior was matching up with my intentions sounded like it could make life easier, and in fact it has.

To begin, take out a piece of paper (sure, the computer will work, but writing things on paper just feels more important and permanent, doesn't it?) and create a list of keywords that sum you up, or at least that sum up your truest interests. In this process you need to dig deep to find out what core values you hold, as opposed to the ones you feel others think you should have, or even those you think you should have.

My (and my family's) keywords were nature, strength, nourishment, clean, sustainable, service, community, efficacy, fun, laughter, experimentation, discovery, play, challenge, wonder.

From there, we clarified what it is about each term that was really calling us. For example, nature is great, but I don't really find looking at it as stimulating as moving through it. So we expanded each word into a sentence fragment: moving through nature, constantly improving strength, being of service to others…you get the idea.

Then we started stacking these phrases to see where there was overlap. We want to experiment with how moving through nature changes how we grow stronger. We want to be of service to others and build a community by taking others along with us as we experiment with growing stronger while moving through nature, reducing our consumption, and cracking up as we fall and learn how to do it better. I'm not going to include my family's final mission statement here, as it's a small treasure we keep amongst the four of us, but we continued with this process of stacking statements until we had one that really stated our purpose as a family.

Once you've got your mission statement, I encourage you to constantly check back in; you'll find you and your priorities change as you change how you move. It's likely your mission (and thus statement) will refine over time and you might find, as we did, that the better your statement represents the realest you, the easier you will find stacking your life.

For example, I value both work-free time and time with my partner and community. However, I had so little time that I kept putting movement into my free-time slot (I really love to exercise), which left less couple time than I wanted. When I compared our regular date activity to our mission statement, I found that "date night"—time my husband and I had set aside for ourselves as a couple—was typically spent doing things we didn't feel passionate about. No, I'm not talking about each other! I mean that even though going to a movie or out to a long dinner was amazing and nourishing, it wasn't really "us." So we came up with "date hike." Once we realized that going out to a fancy place, or even going out at night, really wasn't central to our connection, everything else fell into place.

Date hikes give us a few uninterrupted daylight hours—frankly, when we're both at our best anyway—to move through nature, to sometimes end up at a hot spring, to have long, uninterrupted conversations, to go to places we've never been before. And did I mention it was way easier to find someone to watch the kids during the day? Our kids get to spend some daylight hours— frankly, when they're at their best too—playing with other people who love them. We all felt better after transitioning from date night to date hike, and my husband and I feel refreshed and invigorated—better nourished—by our date time together. (And, P.S., sometimes we still just choose a restaurant or bar that serves fresh, local food and play Scrabble and have a whiskey because that's stacking your life as well.)

My mission statement also helps keep my personal battle with sedentarism in check. (Truly, I'm as sedentary-natured as the next person, I just work on it all the time, constantly, never-endingly, really a lot.) Once a week the kids take a ninety-minute French class at an "indoor school," as my son calls it (isn't perspective amazing?) not too far from their outdoor school site. Typically I've already walked five miles in the early morning and while doing work errands throughout the day, and the kids have been at nature school for four hours, so we pick them up to eat, then drive back to their class in the hour-long break between schools. One day my husband said, "Let's pack lunch and walk to French." And I resisted, because I'd already walked (like, I'd met my daily need) and I was settled in and cozy (by which I mean I was sedentary and loving it), and was thinking (or is it projecting?) that the kids would want to—need to, even—come in and relax after being outside all morning. But I agreed to do it anyway because the mission statement revealed it was a good decision. With the mission statement's assistance, I see that my desire to not move is my deal, and not my husband's or the kids'.

Long story short, everyone, including me, was stoked to eat our lunch as we took the forty-five minute, mile-and-a-half walk to French class. And here's the aha moment: What I normally have to deal with every day—the crankiness that comes with transitioning from school to home, and all the buckling, and close proximity, noise, and stress, and JUST GET IN YOUR SEAT!—didn't happen.

My husband's crazy idea sounded like it was going to be too much work (because deep down that's always my reaction, even if that's not the words I put to it), but it turns out it was just work of a different kind. I could stay inside and drive and "rest" and do the same amount of work via muscle tension and stress hormones and keeping my cool, or I could do it with my legs, arms, and core, and so could the kids.

Your mission statement is probably going to have you getting up and going outside more often, walking to whatever your version of that French class is. Certainly having to do all the wrestling of tiny bodies is also work, but hear this: If you have kids, you're going to do the work either way. And you don't have to have small kids to wrestle with a lack of motivation; there's plenty of work to do to overcome that in every individual. I have yet to encounter an instance when I (and all the other people in my family) don't feel better after choosing to do more physically challenging work. What if there is no "easier," and there is only "less movement?" Now there's something to think about!

When it comes to mission statements, I wouldn't presume that you do or should hold the same core values as I. For example, I am not an artistic person, but I imagine if you were, "create" might be a keyword on your starting list. The great news is, everything comes from nature, which means everyone can find a portal to their needs that honors all of our nature—the natural need to move and our natural constitution and personal ways of finding joy. I do believe that all of us can, to the best of our abilities, execute our lives in a way that matches the values we each hold.

If your values and execution don't match—if your life is not as nourishing as it could be—I'd suggest you take a closer look at yourself. You might hold different, deeper values that have yet to be consciously fleshed out (in which case, revisit your keywords and phrases to see what's missing, or what might need to be removed from your list). Or maybe you're not considering your personal core values when deciding upon which tasks to execute (can you get your mission statement tattooed somewhere easy to reference?). Or perhaps you simply haven't yet discovered the tasks that fit your life well (which to me is the most exciting, wondrous, active part of stacking—the search!).

As I've already said, a mission statement isn't going to reduce the work you have to do. Life is always work of some kind or another.

In fact, you'll probably find that following a personal mission statement makes you work harder, just in the direction you have decided you want to go.

ELDERBERRY

I recently harvested an entire bucket of elderberries to make cough syrup. I was forty years old before I'd ever heard about elderberry syrup, and none of my friends or family had ever made it before; I only just learned about its use in traditional medicine during a wild medicine class. I read up online about the different kinds of elderberry plants and how to make syrup, and I read various research papers (of course) on its effectiveness.

While I was reaching and stretching and climbing trees to gather the berries from various sources, I kept thinking about how the process of gathering them, too, might be influencing my total well-being. The work to gather, performed by my arms and legs, my hips, shoulders, and hands, and all the parts in between, kept me moving. My kids and my nieces and nephews were there in the sun—and natural light, open space, fresh air, and dirt—gathering with me, which meant I was providing fellow parents with child-care *and* moving the kids, so those of us there and not there were benefitting from precious family and community time. As the kids and I reached and squatted and scampered over to eat from the blackberry bushes that also surrounded us, I passed on the information I had previously gathered on elderberries (which, again, I learned from the internet—thanks, internet!). As we observed the plants and their various parts, we started noticing other things, like that certain birds flew in to inspect the tops of the bushes we were gathering from, and how the chickens were watching what we were doing and soon arrived at our feet to gobble up the berries we'd dislodged while gathering. I imagine that had we been doing this year after year, decade after decade, we'd have a better sense of where elderberry time fell along the timelines for harvesting other plants, and how certain weather patterns made for years with few elderberries, and some for the abundance we were met with on this day.

I had plenty of time to think about this as we squatted to pull the berries, cook them for a bit (can you imagine the work I would have had to do if I didn't have a pot, a stove, and running water in my house?), and mash them through a sieve into what eventually became elderberry syrup.

The extract of elderberry is helpful—I've seen all that research—but as I was gathering I was wondering how the benefit of the extract compares to the benefit of the entire syrup-making process.

I've always had a strong need to understand nature. But rather than continuing to simply wonder—if more parts of this phenomenon of elderberry syrup will ever be researched; when more parts of health and human science will be understood; whose responsibility it is to integrate them all; and whose job it is to relay the whole picture to everyone else—I'm taking action.

I've recently become aware that one of the greatest unstackings of my life, personally, was how I was meeting my need to know nature. For decades I'd been trying to meet this need through thousands of hours of research and reading and questioning and writing—to the detriment of many of my other needs. Then I found that I could meet my need to understand through the regular practice of getting to know nature with my body. I can pick and process elderberries to learn which movements it takes. I can spend time with a community of people in nature to see how it shapes them. What gathering elderberries provides, beyond the extract, is a fully stacked experience of my body and mind. These experiences have facilitated the understanding that I, too, am nature, and for that reason I am efficient. I just had to get beyond the parts in my mind to understand. I had to get moving to prove it to myself, naturally.

DEAR KATY

Q WHAT IN YOUR OPINION IS THE IMPLICATION FOR US—AS A SPECIES—OF NOT MOVING TO OUR FULL CAPABILITIES?

A Science defines humanness by genetics, morphology (our structural features), and behavior—and how these compare to all other living things. I think the way the bulk of us have been moving as a species has perpetuated changes to the morphology of *certain* human groups, and that our lack of motion is transitioning us toward, by our own classification system, a functionally domesticated version of a human—one no longer able to reproduce and survive without major technological interventions and the work of other humans to provide us life support.

Human domestication is expensive. If you took the time to calculate the cost of all the movement that is outsourced for one "domesticated" human to survive for ten years, you'd likely find the cost exorbitant—especially in fossil fuel and in wilderness. For those reasons, human movement as we've been doing it for the last few hundred years (which is hardly any time at all) is unsustainable for the future of our species. I would say the bulk of modern human animals are moving (or is it unmoving?) towards there being fewer total humans in the long run.

Q IT FEELS LIKE "STACKING YOUR LIFE" IS MOST EASILY DONE
IN A RURAL AREA. HOW CAN SOMEONE STACK IF THEY
LIVE IN A LARGE URBAN AREA? HOW EXPENSIVE IS IT? AND
WHAT ABOUT SINGLE PARENTS WORKING TWO JOBS WHO
CAN'T FIND ANY EXTRA TIME?

A When it comes to the seeming impossibility of stacking, I receive
just as many emails from my rural readers about the difficulty of
accomplishing this lifestyle when isolated out in the wilderness
as I do from urbanites. Where you live simply offers a different
launching point; no place or situation limits your progress as
much as it sets a different stage.

The bonuses of an urban landscape include more people with
whom to build a community, more built-in walking to errands
and jobs and visits, and more options when it comes to stores
and restaurants and farmers' markets. And did you know there are
even wild food foraging groups in New York City, Los Angeles,
and San Francisco? I know it seems like plants aren't abundant in
these areas, but they are there. The problem is rarely one of availability, but of knowledge.

The best place to start is with an internet search on your local
area. Make a list of any adult or child nature programs, foraging
classes, traditional food preparation, permaculture, bushcraft
classes, or gleaning groups in your area.

Depending on where you live, classes can get expensive. If you've
already cut many nonessentials and are still struggling to afford
your life, watch for free or inexpensive community-building

events and offer to volunteer or assist with a course in lieu of paying for it, or barter your services/skill set. Inquire about scholarships, or if you're in the position to, donate to programs or provide scholarship funding that will benefit someone in your local community.

Most likely there are other people in your area working hard, just like you, at building communities that bring them closer to some of the ideas in this book. The ideas in this book—the need for others, the maintenance of traditional skills, permaculture—aren't novel, I've just related them all back to sedentarism. Meaning, it's likely you don't have to start something from scratch, but rather simply find and join. No matter the specifics of your current home dynamic, you and your family have something to offer these groups and they you—you just have to clarify the details of your symbiosis.

We are used to the things that improve our health costing more and taking additional time, but when it comes to stacking, you're often wasting less time and money. A minimal/maximal lifestyle largely comprises inexpensive behaviors that get you moving. Foraging, walking, and forgoing furniture are often available to you for no money. Also, more and more cities are developing urban farms[23] to improve food rights in low-income communities, and one way to stack your life is to get involved with one near you.

If you're struggling to find time—if you're a single parent with two jobs—then community really is key. My own single, full-time-working mother moved us to a rural area that cost less and where we could be closer to family members that could help. (This is actually how I ended up working on a family farm at such a young age.) I think we keep focusing on the traditional family unit as the only way to stack (you'll be stacked once your family looks "normal"), but the *real* traditional unit is a group of people of multiple generations, some with children and some without. Looking to these others as another way of stacking your life for better support and more movement opens many more options.

To those readers already nourished with community and some flexibility when it comes to how you can stack, you can move to seek out members of your community who are struggling and offer to help them in a way that helps both of you stack: take their children along with you on a foraging walk (more kids on a walk makes it easier, I've discovered, over and over again); invite them to a once-a-week or once-a-month soup night or picnic in a park; offer to pick up their groceries when you walk out for yours.

When you're new to stacking, a phase that can last years, the most challenging part isn't necessarily where and how you're currently living, but rather changing the way you think about how to meet your needs. Whether you're rural or urban, your movement can be of direct help to someone else in your community, but this is a symbiosis, remember? You're being helped as you're helping, and you stacking brings others into a more stacked place. Everyone benefits when your life is stacked, which is why the work to stack it might be some of the most meaningful, impactful work you can do.

Q I'VE JUST READ [AN ADVANCE COPY OF] THIS BOOK AND
IT'S KIND OF FREAKING ME OUT HOW JUST LIVING MY
LIFE IN A PEACEFUL WAY (AS I'VE PERCEIVED IT) COULD BE
CONTRIBUTING TO ALL THE WORLD'S PROBLEMS. WHERE
DO I GO FROM HERE? RIGHT NOW, I'M FEELING OVER-
WHELMED.

A You can view the message of this book in a couple of ways.
The first is to recognize how much you've been outsourcing
movement and feel terrible about it. The second is to see all the
ways in which you've been outsourcing movement as endless
opportunities to make a direct, positive improvement in the
world through personal action that also entirely benefits you. I
focus on the latter perspective for obvious reasons, but also for
a not-as-obvious one: A lot of people want to make the world
a better place and perhaps have seen "make the world a better
place" as another obligation to add to their out-of-control to-do
list. Contributing positively to the world is often viewed as
something to do with our extra time or money. But most of us
don't have large amounts of extra time or money. We're barely
meeting our own needs, and so our ability to contribute largely
to the improvement of many problems is small. And the fact of
the matter is, in our constant struggle to meet our personal needs
we're often working against the very things we value.

What an easy solution then: You need to move and the world
needs you to move and the ways you can start moving more on
your own behalf are so numerous that you can really start with
any of the examples I've used in this book. Start by turning your

car key instead of using a battery-powered clicker to open your car doors, and forgo teabags in favor of loose tea; walk instead of driving; buy local food; source raw ingredients and process them yourself; process some of them manually; learn some local wild foods or grow a few plants in your yard; buy handmade items from those making them for a wage and under a set of conditions you deem acceptable; take care of your body by choosing exercises designed to improve and maintain your whole-body function over time; volunteer some of your exercise time and spend it at a local farm, squatting to weed or harvest; take a class or find a mentor that will help you develop nature competency so you can make going outside in nature a hobby; eat outside; eat inside, but on the floor; start a community soup night; move with others who are less able and need assistance; start a walking book group; start paying attention to how you move, how much you move, and especially how much you don't.

Question everything, including what you're doing right this minute and what has made what you're doing possible. Just so you know, this book was printed in the United States on recycled paper, and it was written, edited, designed, edited again, and again, and again, and marketed, all by individuals who made personal choices to leave their traditional office jobs in publishing houses and media to freelance from home to better meet their personal needs and the needs of their personal ecosystems. They've stacked their lives, and choosing to work with these individuals rather than their more conventional (less stacked) counterparts is another way I've stacked my life and improved my own personal ecosystem. Also, a note on the carrot pictures on pages 95 and 96 from the essay "Those Other Nutrients": My kids and I grew those carrots in our backyard; the kids pulled and washed them while I was writing parts of this book; my husband took the pictures; and the tools from our kitchen in the photos— the grater, the cutting board, the knife, and the baking dish— were all purchased at garage sales. This picture is "stack your life" personified. Or I guess it's picturefied. Either way, now you know a little more about how what you've chosen to do right now, which is read this book, came to be possible.

P.S. This is only my second year growing a garden. The first year, I grew eleven toothpick-sized carrots; this year I got one baking dish full of medium-sized carrots. I'm *transitioning* to becoming someone who grows things, friends. It's going to take a long, long time for my yields to match my passion, but I don't feel like I'm failing until I nail it. I figure I started nailing it when I chose to try.

---

23. Visit urbanfarming.org for more information.

AFTERWORD
AND ACKNOWLEDGMENTS

I didn't set out to write a book on movement activism, sedentary culture, and the cost of our nature deficit. *Movement Matters* was initially proposed as a collection of blog posts and other articles I wrote between 2012 and 2016, in the style of *Alignment Matters,* a collection of the first five years of my attempt to teach the basics of alignment via my blog. My editor gathered some of the most powerful pieces and sent them to me for a read-through, minor edits, and my input on how they should be organized into sections.

As I read, it quickly became clear to me that the essays were disjointed. My blog has served as a way to blurt out the initial thoughts that pass through my head whenever some sort of input—a research article, a headline, a passage in a book, a line from a song—stimulates something in my mind. And so the articles she assembled were just a series of shouts off the top of my head, and I wasn't particularly inspired to organize them in any way.

I decided to take a few days away from my computer, my work, and my home to go camping with my family and clear my mind. We hadn't even been in the woods for a full day when it hit me— each of my posts or articles had touched on a random aspect of the same essential problem: that we are a sedentary culture and our lack of movement affects our thoughts, which in turn reinforces our sedentarism. I had never noticed the underlying premise of all of my short "essays," because I was too busy blurting out posts on my blog. But as I read through all of them again, there it was—that common idea buried within almost everything I'd written over the last few years: we move how we think.

Instead of a light edit, most articles needed a complete rewrite to speak more directly to the newly identified theme. I adjusted the details of the essays one by one to better address the book's focus. But about two-thirds of the way through, I lost sight of where I was going with this collection. Luckily, I was heading out to trek the Southwest, where I'd be walking through parts of the world that are still similar to how they were thousands of years ago, largely thanks to our National Parks system. I anticipated that being immersed in nature would once again help me to engage with the material. It was while I was flying there, however, that I received my next inspiration.

Looking at the planet from thirty thousand feet up offers a different perspective from the usual. (I took note when Marc Reisner, in the introduction to *Cadillac Desert,* pointed out that "anyone who flies in an airplane and doesn't spend most of his time looking out the window wastes his money.") Looking at the winding rivers from far above, and how their water has etched their mark into the crust of the earth, I thought about the relationship between humans and water and dams.

So many humans are well-practiced in casting. Sometimes realizing it and sometimes not, we've limited the motion of our bodies, limited the motion of many other human and non-human animals, and we've also significantly limited the motion of other natural things, like rivers.

A river, if allowed to move freely, changes its course over time, and distributes the result of its movement over a broader area. A dammed river creates a sort of repetitive-use injury on the planet. Our "casted" culture has casted most rivers, changing how and where they move, and where they don't move, which in turn changes the soils and plants and animals around them. Looking at the planet from above made me wonder: Did we cast our bodies first and then turn our attention to larger casting behaviors, or was it the other way around; did we try to cast the big things in nature and, as a result, wind up in a cast? Or did they happen in lockstep, initiated by something else?

These are the types of thoughts I have when surrounded by the results of a billion years of movement, in a body itself fashioned and maintained by a long history of movement. By immersing myself and my thoughts in wildly natural places, the seeds of these thoughts were nourished, and grew into my final essays. I had seen research on this before—that time spent immersed in nature boosted creativity[1]—but I hadn't, until then, lived out the experiment myself.

It is not lost on me that what it took for me to write this book was to live, at least in part, what this book is about. And as I lived it, more words came (the entire fourth section was written just for this book; none of those essays were part of the original essays compiled by my editor). By the time I reached the end, I was even more inspired to shift our family's actions *even more* in line with ideas contained in this book. It's a strange phenomenon I won't even try to explain, but I've experienced reading and learning from these essays as if they were written by someone other than me.

I was not outdoorsy nor even a mover growing up. While we did have a small farm, I am not from a family that engaged regularly in nature. I do not have a history of loving the great outdoors, and I've always been most comfortable sitting and reading book after book after book. Looking back, I can see that my transition to being a mover who prioritizes nature and outdoor experience every day came about via a cycle of insight, research, insight, research, insight, research. After being inspired, I'd turn to academia to make sense of an insight in the hopes that what I should do would become clear. In the end I remembered science does not tell you what to do with the facts its process has revealed—the integration and application of facts comes from within, passing through our personal perceptions of how the world works.

I've always felt rich in knowledge, but what I didn't understand before, what wasn't made clear to me throughout my training, is that knowledge isn't wisdom. Knowledge is an awareness of facts, nothing more; just knowing something doesn't tell you how to apply these facts to your life, or how these facts relate to all other facts, or to life. I currently live in a happy place between regularly using the scientific process for knowledge while understanding how knowledge relates to wisdom; the final decision on how to behave lies with each of us alone, and science does not have an opinion on the matter. For me, insights are the roots, wisdom is the tree, and knowledge is the air, water, and sunlight. The seeds of a tree are the mechanism of sharing—easily distributed parts that can grow, for each person, into a unique shape that depends on the individual doing the growing.

In academia, it's common to note whose work has informed your own. You can see the references and writings as they're noted in each essay in this book, but also integral to the ideas contained in *Movement Matters* are books I happened upon that were seemingly unrelated, yet critical to the theses I work on every day. These books facilitated insights that functioned either as a fastener between previously unattached ideas or a breadcrumb toward something new. In the order I read them, they are: *Cadillac Desert* by Marc Reisner; *The Final Forest* by William Dietrich; *The Unlikely Peace at Cuchumaquic* by Martin Prechtel; *Colonialism & Science* by James E. McClellan III; *Leaving Before the Rains Come* by Alexandra Fuller; *The Navajo and the Animal People* by Steve Pavlik; *On Growth and Form* by D'Arcy Wentworth Thompson; the entire Hatchet series by Gary Paulsen; and *So Human an Animal* and *Man Adapting* by René Dubos.

Passages within these books, in addition to every other book I've read, every course I've ever taken, every conversation I've ever had, every Facebook comment I've ever read, and every moment spent engaging with my children, have led me to the content presented in *Movement Matters*.

I'm additionally inspired, regularly, by a handful of people and the contribution they're putting forth with their life-time: Sarah Salazar-Tipton, Erwan and Jessika Le Corre, Sam Thayer, Arthur Haines, Daniel Vitalis, Diana Rodgers, Ashley Judd, and Richard Louv.

The people I work with on a daily basis, or rather, those whose gifts seem to make my work more clear, more palatable, and a better reflection of my most authentic self: Penelope Jackson, Zsofi Koller, Kate Kennedy, Agnes Koller, Debbie Beane, Dani Hemmat, Stephanie Domet, and Penelope Jackson again.

To those who have gifted their time in discussing and reviewing various portions of this manuscript: Richard Ollerton, PhD, mathematician extraordinaire, Dr. Jeannette Loram and Dr. Jessica Worthington Wilmer, biologists supreme, and Barbara L. Reiss, OD (for her review as well as ongoing discussions on myopia and eye mechanics!).

This book would not have been written if I didn't have the most faithful walking buddy of all time, so miles and miles of thanks to Jordan Schiefen.

This book would not have been written if it weren't for the people who so generously love and care for my children, especially my mother and sister, as well as the rest of my family, my tribe, my flock.

The soundtrack for this book was every song performed by the Eagles. RIP Glenn Frey, and thanks for all the good times.

Without the people listed here, I am simply a lone goose beating her wings, fatiguing in the wind and going nowhere, but there has never been a lead goose with as much stamina as you, Michael Curran. Moving into your flock was the best "stack your life" decision I've ever made.

---

1. Atchley, Ruth Ann, David L. Strayer, and Paul Atchley. 2012. "Creativity in the Wild: Improving Creative Reasoning through Immersion in Natural Settings." *PLoS ONE* 7(12): e51474. doi:10.1371/journal.pone.0051474.

APPENDICES

APPENDIX 1: NATURE IN EDUCATION

It's been shown over and over again through research (look at the trove here: childrenandnature.org/learn/news-center) and through parents' own experiences that children do well with a hefty amount of time outside in nature, whether it's at home and in the community, as part of traditional schooling, or in nature school. Where and how we live can affect the nature opportunities available to us, but fortunately, experts have already considered these limitations and provided various ways of making more nature in education a reality. Many thanks to Sarah Salazar-Tipton, the director of our local "reconnect with nature" organization, for her help in compiling these resources!

BRING MORE NATURE TO YOUR HOME AND COMMUNITY

- **Nature-scape your backyard**. Consider opening up your backyard to your community or neighborhood so that children know they can come by and play whenever they want, or at certain hours. Find tips at: modernparentsmessykids.com/2012/05/how-to-set-up-natural-play-spaces-in.html.
- **Join or start a community nature group**, like a wildcrafting or tracking group, in which you can gather to learn about nature and how to read the landscape to tell the stories of what is going on with animals and plants. One great example is set up by the p.i.n.e. project; check it out at: pineproject.org/program/tracking-and-nature-club.
- **Join or start a family hiking, camping, or play group**, where families can get together to play, hike, or explore. To find a program

in your area or see examples of programs you could emulate, search "family drop-in nature programs."

BRING MORE NATURE TO SCHOOL

- **Check out author Herbert Broda**, who writes books about bringing more nature into the classroom and bringing the class out into nature. Look for his books *Schoolyard-Enhanced Learning* and *Moving the Classroom Outdoors.*
- **Create a more natural playspace** at your children's school. See the natural playscape link in the previous section, or create simple changes such as leaving an area of grass unmowed, maintaining bird feeders, and introducing more trees and shrubs.
- **Create a school garden** so children can connect directly with natural cycles and spend quality educational time outside.
- **Set up field trips to Audubon or other nature centers**. Our local Audubon center hosts every child in our county for a day-long science field trip when the kids are in the fifth grade. They conduct actual science experiments that help the center determine the fish habitat quality.

ATTEND OR START A NATURE SCHOOL

Nature preschools and forest kindergartens are becoming increasingly popular. As with any school, there are many variations—non-profit or for profit, curriculum or no curriculum, partially or completely outdoors, teacher to student ratios, etc. More rare but growing are elementary-school programs. My children's nature school began as a preschool, but as the enrolled children get older, the program is being expanded. Nature school doesn't have to be all-or-nothing; you could run an after-school or weekend program for school-aged kids, or a half-day preschool completely centered in nature.

If you are interested in becoming a nature school instructor yourself, there are many ways to go about it. Training for nature-based education is varied and can come through traditional avenues like university or community college (outdoor education or experiential education degrees), naturalist study programs and certificates, or early childhood education degrees.

RESOURCES

- **Wilderness Awareness School** has an excellent weekend and week-long program on mentoring children in nature called Coyote Mentoring. Check out wildernessawareness.org/adult/coyote-mentoring.
- **Authors** David Sobel (*Childhood and Nature, Place-Based Education, Mapmaking with Children*), Erin Kenny (*Forest Kindergartens the Cedarsong Way*), and Karen Constable (*The Outdoor Classroom Ages 3–7*) have all written excellent resources for nature educators.
- **Local non-profits or nature centers** may be interested in partnering with you. Start your search at Natural Start Alliance (naturalstart.org) and the Children and Nature Network (childrenandnature.org/connect).
- *Coyote's Guide to Connecting with Nature* by Jon Young, Evan McGown, and Ellen Haas is an excellent resource, no matter how you wish to integrate more nature into your life.

APPENDIX 2: FORAGING

Foraging has become a hobby for those who can easily buy food at the store, but it's important to remember that it's the way many people subsist on the planet today, and how all people used to subsist. You can approach foraging from many angles: as a fun hobby, as a way of maintaining a potentially necessary skill in the natural world, and as one way to address many of the problems—physical, social, economical, environmental—we wrestle with each day.

If you're new to foraging, here are two sound pieces of advice: Start your foraging in the easy zone (e.g., local fruit trees, abandoned or overgrown gardens) and forage responsibly. Responsible foraging, as taught by the nature school in my area, follows the one-third rule: harvest one-third of a plant's offerings for yourself, leaving one-third for other animals and the other third for the plants.

Beyond basic guidelines on quantities, there are more complex principles of wild harvest. Robin Wall Kimmerer, a professor of environmental and forest biology, describes these in *Braiding Sweetgrass: Indigenous Wisdom, Scientific Knowledge, and the Teachings of Plants.* In the Winter 2016 issue of *Yes Magazine*, Kimmerer names food gathering the "Honorable Harvest" and describes it as a "canon of indigenous principles that govern the exchange of life for life" that is "both ancient and urgent." The primary theme to her list of principles is that it is not specifically about the quantities you take, but the bigger picture of taking in general: "Sustain the ones who sustain you, and the Earth will last forever." Whichever guideline you hold in the front of your mind, here are some simple ways you can begin foraging:

- **Start with the familiar.** Begin your foraging journey with what you already know. Have you ever walked past an apple, orange, or pear that has fallen to the sidewalk, destined to rot? Change that fruit's destiny, and pick it up! (And by bending and squatting down to do so, you may adjust a little bit of your own destiny too!)

- **Be neighborly.** Before I moved to Washington, I lived in Southern California—a.k.a. the land of houses with avocado and citrus trees in almost every yard, avocado and citrus rotting under those trees, and fridges full of imported produce. My husband introduced himself to a neighbor with an abundant lemon tree and struck a deal to harvest as many lemons as he wanted as long as he occasionally brought back some lemon curd and lemonade. Now in the Pacific Northwest, we often find fruit trees that are neglected and lousy with food. We don't only harvest for ourselves—we'll approach neighbors too frail to gather their own fruit and harvest for them. In this way we move, gather food, spend family time together, and strengthen our community all at once—some serious stacking in action. There are also many "gleaning" organizations that list unpicked food going to waste and ask for volunteers to pick that food for local food banks. Search "gleaning" and the name of your local area to see how you can participate.

- **Get the kids involved.** My family has a list of easy-to-find wild edibles to keep our foraging chops well-practiced. Herbs like rosemary, lemon balm, and lemongrass are abundant in our neighborhood, as are dandelions and nettle. I send the kids out for something for every meal even if I don't really need it. I want them to associate moving their bodies outside, if only for a few minutes, with contributing to the family meal. And sometimes we'll make herbal tea just because, and the kids love experimenting with tea flavors.

- **Take a local class or workshop.** Check in with your local Audubon Center, natural foods market, community boards, or newspapers. There are a lot of people passionate about using the stuff growing in the public nature areas nearby, and eager to share their passion and knowledge.
- **Get a guide—a person or a book.** You may meet that guide at the workshop you just attended (see how that works!). Also, there are plenty of books available on wild edibles. Pick the one that seems like it'd be easiest to use. Just make sure it focuses on your geographical region.
- **Search your favorite author on YouTube.** If only Sam Thayer lived in my neighborhood so he could teach me something…Oh wait, here he is in my computer! It is an amazing time to be alive, isn't it?

Sam Thayer is my foraging guru and my favorite guide is his book *Forager's Harvest*. A lot of foraging books are quite dry (here's the plant, how to identify, how to not confuse it with a potentially harmful one, etc.), but his book is full of easy-to-digest, entertaining stories that make you think of both the details and the broader picture differently. The section on acorns is worth the purchase price alone; it describes how the bias of plant science went along with the racist biases of the people from the time the plant science was performed—it was believed that if "natives" were eating something, such as acorns, that food should be thought of as inappropriate or even harmful to "non-natives": "To members of the Fore tribe, [Westerners not sharing in the mushrooms they ate for poisoning fears] probably sounded about as absurd as 'let's not eat these bananas; perhaps they are deadly false bananas' would sound to us."

Thayer refers to what he calls the "Poisonous Plant Fable," laying out many examples of how we have been culturally trained to regard foraging as an inherently dangerous activity. Wild food is not inherently dangerous to humans. Humans have persisted throughout time by foraging. Our current lack of knowledge regarding wild food sources is definitely a challenge, but when guided by someone rich in plant wisdom, wild plant gathering is inherently delightful, fun, and fulfilling—pun intended.

APPENDIX 3: BREASTFEEDING

There's a lot of "breast-is-best" mentality out there that, right off the bat, can make many people who are unable or choosing not to breastfeed feel badly. Instead of contributing to that perspective, I prefer a more scientific approach and the "breast-is-breast" message.

A breast-is-breast perspective is one that seeks answers to questions like "How do breasts and breast milk and breastfeeding work?" Instead of starting with the assumption that all methods of feeding a baby are equal (similar to how much of our science assumes that walking over terrain is the same as walking on a treadmill; see the essay "Proof" on page 26), the breast-is-breast mentality calls for specific definitions and investigations. We all have to make decisions about our own lives, and the more information we have, the more we can ensure our decisions align with our personal mission statements.

"Breast is breast" is also "bottle fed is bottle fed" is also "bottle delivered breast milk previously frozen is bottle delivered breast milk previously frozen" is also "bottle delivered formula is bottle delivered formula." This approach allows us to be more specific in our investigation and to consider the largest perspective possible when we're gathering data, so we can accurately represent and assess the details. When you read research or opinion pieces on feeding babies, always check to see how breast and bottle feeding are defined when weighing the conclusions at hand.

If you're interested in information on the culture and history of our and other cultures' relationships with breastfeeding, here are some resources to check out:

- *Lactivism: How Feminists and Fundamentalists, Hippies and Yuppies, and Physicians and Politicians Made Breastfeeding Big Business and Bad Policy* by Courtney Jung. In the *New York Times*, Lori Gottlieb writes of this book: "Perhaps most interesting is Jung's astute observation that what is being so ardently promoted isn't actual breast-feeding—whereby a baby is fed from the breast—but human milk as a product, creating pressure for working mothers of all income levels to pump in less than ideal conditions, when what might benefit them and their babies most is paid maternity leave." This delineation and the critical lens with which Jung views the cultural context of breastfeeding are essential reading.
- **kathydettwyler.weebly.com**. Kathy Dettwyler is an anthropologist who offers an abundance of research regarding worldwide breastfeeding practices on her website. See also the book she co-edited with Patricia Stuart-Macadam, *Breastfeeding: Biocultural Perspectives*.
- *Hunter-Gatherer Childhoods: Evolutionary, Developmental, and Cultural Perspectives,* edited by Michael E. Lamb and Barry S. Hewlett. The book is a compendium of literature describing various childhood practices, and it is the best source for valuable insight into the varying breastfeeding practices found in certain hunter-gatherer cultures.

If you're interested in breastfeeding and want in-person assistance or support, there are groups and services available. You can contact your local hospital or nursing group to request an appointment with a lactation consultant, hire a postpartum doula, or meet up with your local La Leche League or other breastfeeding support group.

Websites offering support:

- La Leche League: llli.org
- KellyMom: kellymom.com
- International Breastfeeding Centre: nbci.ca

INDEX

A

activism, 196–198

addiction, 178–180

Alignment Matters (book), by Katy Bowman, 4

ankles, 24, 52–53, 65, 80, 139, 161

anthropology, 4, 22, 58, 214

anxiety, 46, 178

apples, 98–99, 113–114, 210

athletics, 90, 116, 152

B

baby-carrying, 6, 153–154

bacteria, 74–76, 101, 145, 172

Bateson, Gregory, 88

bees, *see* honeybee

bicycles, *see* cycling

birthing, 21–22

Blood and Earth: Modern Slavery, Ecocide, and the Secret to Saving the World (book), by Kevin Bales, 111

blood vessels, 18–19, 48, 66

Boeing, 153

bone density, 62–63

brain, human,

    shape, 52

    lymph, 128

breastfeeding, 99–103, 124, 167, 213–215

Brenoff, Ann, 35

bugs, 50, 79, 142, 145

Bureau of International Labor Affairs, 110

C

Cadillac Desert (book), by Marc Reisner, 200, 203

calories, 26, 73-77, 99, 111, 125, 126, 144, 166

carbon footprint, 126-127

carrots, 95-96, 198

casts, 200-201

cell phones, *see* mobile phones

cellular biology, 37

chewing, 92-96, 101, 114, 117, 144

child labor, *see* forced labor

childbirth, 21-25

chocolate, 110, 118

choices, 9, 35, 41, 47, 56, 77, 85, 112, 137, 197

climbing trees, 50-54, 91, 106, 156, 189

Clinical Anatomy Made Ridiculously Simple (book), by Stephen Goldberg, 65

commodity, 115-117

cough syrup, 189

counter-culture, 163-168

cycling, 57, 153

D

da Vinci, Leonardo, 57

dance, 116, 152

Daniel, Thomas, 18

delineation, 68-70, 101, 179, 214

depression, 46, 178-181

Dettwyler, Kathy (anthropologist), 214

disabilities, 4, 118-119

distance-looking, 65-70, 119

domestication (of humans), 192

dorsiflexion, 52-53

H

Hales, T.C., 138

Harvard Health Publications (a division of Harvard Medical
      School), 144-145, 149

hiking,
      kids, 55-56, 206
      date hike, 185

honeybee, 1, 134-136, 175

Huffington Post, 35

The Human Body (book), by Jonathan Miller, 17

The Human Machine (book), by George B. Bridgman, 92-94

human trafficking, *see* forced labor

hunger, xxi, 56, 88, 151

hydroxyapatite, 63

I

Ill Nature (book), by Joy Williams, 29

indoors, 59, 69-71, 171, 185

informed, staying, 40, 46

insects, *see* bugs

J

Journal of Obesity Research and Clinical Practice, 73-78

joy, 161-162, 187

Judd, Ashley, 7, 203

Juvenal, 124

K

key fob, 9

kids hiking, *see* hiking, kids

kinesiology, 6, 152

Kondo, Marie, 139

osteoporosis/osteoarthritis, 26, 59, 77, 94, 147
outdoor school, 79-81, 107, 185, 206-208
outliers, 155, 166
outsourcing of movement, 9, 88-89, 92-94, 98, 101-102, 106,
     109-117, 127, 159, 177, 192, 196
ovum, *see* egg
Oxford Junior Dictionary, 72-73, 76

P

pain, xix, 3-5, 94, 157, 160, 178-179
parts of a whole, 13, 19-25, 37, 126, 128-133, 134, 142-143, 146,
     148-149, 158-160, 171-172, 177, 189-190
paths, xx, 55-56, 83-85
pelvic floor, 27, 171
permaculture, 107-108, 193-194
Petrie, Ryan, 38
Playfair, John, 44
Pobjoy, Ben, xvii–xxii
Pollan, Michael, 166-167
pollution, 30, 74-76
processed/processing food, 84, 90-97, 111, 117, 131, 143-147,
     158, 176, 189-190, 197
proof, 6, 26-31, 33, 40, 127, 142, 213

R

"real world", 120-121
reduction (in science), 6, 37, 46, 76, 79, 128-133,134
rivers, 44, 48-49, 61, 200-201
rural, 193-194

S

school, *see* outdoor school

ScienceDaily, 22

Scully, Jackie Leach (author of paper, "What is a Disease?"), 6

scurvy, 178-179

shock-absorbing goo, *see* hydroxyapatite

shoes, xx, 2, 109, 139

signs, 50-51, 84, 152-154, 169-170, 173

sitting, 35, 65, 68, 79, 112, 120, 147

slave labor, *see* forced labor

Southwest (of United States), 200

stacking/stacked/unstacked, xix, 104-108, 118-120, 128, 134-141, 142, 145, 147-149, 160, 167, 170, 171, 176-178, 181, 184-185

standing, 35, 65

stillness, 4, 37, 65, 109, 116

stupid, 35-36

surgery, 126

sustainability/unsustainability, 47, 83-85, 102, 108, 116, 125, 135, 146, 155, 163, 166, 168, 180-181, 183, 192, 209

T

tea bag, 9

textbooks, 29, 41, 52, 152

therapy, 27, 93, 101, 102, 157, 169-172, 177-180

thigmomorphogenesis, 50-51

trails, *see* paths

treadmills, 3, 6, 26-31, 40, 143, 213

tree climbing, *see* climbing trees

trees, 48-54, 57-63, 69, 91, 106-107, 128-130, 176, 181, 202, 207, 209, 210

Twa, 52-53

U

U.S. Air Force, 153
U.S. Department of Labor, 110
universe, 1-3, 6, 39, 44-46, 121, 181
urbanfarming.org, 198

V

vision, 69-70

W

whole food, 90, 94-96, 98, 113, 130, 142-149, 166
wilderness, 45, 47, 48, 50, 56, 83-85, 116, 156, 192, 193, 208
Williams, David, 18
wisdom, 124, 131, 142, 146, 158, 202, 209, 212

Z

Zinn, Howard, 18
zoos, 6, 169

ABOUT THE AUTHOR

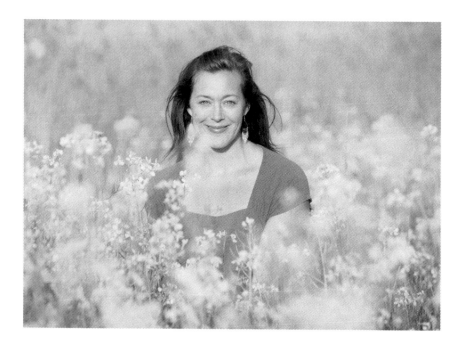

Part biomechanist, part science communicator, and full-time mover, Katy Bowman has educated hundreds of thousands of people on the role movement plays in the body and in the world. Blending a scientific approach with straight talk about sensible, whole-life movement solutions, her website and award-winning podcast, *Katy Says*, reach hundreds of thousands of people every month, and thousands have taken her live classes.

Her books, the bestselling *Move Your DNA* (2014), *Simple Steps to Foot Pain Relief* (2016), *Diastasis Recti* (2016), *Don't Just Sit There* (2015), *Whole Body Barefoot* (2015), *Alignment Matters* (2013), and *Every Woman's Guide to Foot Pain Relief* (2011), have been critically acclaimed and translated worldwide.

Passionate about human movement outside of exercise, Katy volunteers her time to support the larger reintegration of movement into human lives by providing movement courses across widely varying demographics and working with non-profits promoting nature education. She also directs and teaches at the Nutritious Movement™ Center Northwest in Washington state, travels the globe to teach Nutritious Movement courses in person, and spends as much time outside as possible with her husband and children.